Th
Developmentally

Nurturing Wellness in Childhood to Promote Lifelong Health

Andrew S. Garner, MD, PhD, FAAP

Robert A. Saul, MD, FAAP, FACMG

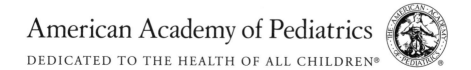

American Academy of Pediatrics
DEDICATED TO THE HEALTH OF ALL CHILDREN®

American Academy of Pediatrics Publishing Staff

Mary Lou White, *Chief Product and Services Officer/SVP, Membership, Marketing, and Publishing*

Mark Grimes, *Vice President, Publishing*

Chris Wiberg, *Senior Editor, Professional/Clinical Publishing*

Theresa Wiener, *Production Manager, Clinical and Professional Publications*

Jason Crase, *Manager, Editorial Services*

Linda Diamond, *Manager, Art Direction and Production*

Sara Hoerdeman, *Marketing Manager, Consumer Products*

345 Park Blvd
Itasca, IL 60143
Telephone: 630/626-6000
Facsimile: 847/434-8000
www.aap.org

The American Academy of Pediatrics is an organization of 66,000 primary care pediatricians, pediatric medical subspecialists, and pediatric surgical specialists dedicated to the health, safety, and well-being of infants, children, adolescents, and young adults.

The recommendations in this publication do not indicate an exclusive course of treatment or serve as a standard of care. Variations, taking into account individual circumstances, may be appropriate.

Statements and opinions expressed are those of the authors and not necessarily those of the American Academy of Pediatrics.

Listing of resources does not imply an endorsement by the American Academy of Pediatrics (AAP). The AAP is not responsible for the content of external resources. Information was current at the time of publication.

Brand names are furnished for identification purposes only. No endorsement of the manufacturers or products mentioned is implied.

The publishers have made every effort to trace the copyright holders for borrowed material. If they have inadvertently overlooked any, they will be pleased to make the necessary arrangements at the first opportunity.

This publication has been developed by the American Academy of Pediatrics. The authors, editors, and contributors are expert authorities in the field of pediatrics. No commercial involvement of any kind has been solicited or accepted in the development of the content of this publication.

Every effort is made to keep *Thinking Developmentally: Nurturing Wellness in Childhood to Promote Lifelong Health* consistent with the most recent advice and information available from the American Academy of Pediatrics.

Special discounts are available for bulk purchases of this publication. E-mail Special Sales at aapsales@aap.org for more information.

Printed in the United States of America

9-407/0919   2 3 4 5 6 7 8 9 10
MA0861
ISBN: 978-1-61002-152-4
eBook: 978-1-61002-153-1
EPUB: 978-1-61002-241-5
Mobi: 978-1-61002-242-2
Cover design by Linda Diamond
Book design by Peg Mulcahy
Library of Congress Control Number: 2017944378

Authors

Andrew S. Garner, MD, PhD, FAAP
Clinical Professor of Pediatrics
Case Western Reserve University School of Medicine
Primary Care Pediatrician
University Hospitals Medical Practices
Cleveland, OH

Robert A. Saul, MD, FAAP, FACMG
Professor of Pediatrics
University of South Carolina School of Medicine Greenville
Medical Director, General Pediatrics Division
Children's Hospital
Greenville Health System
Greenville, SC

American Academy of Pediatrics Reviewers

To all of our families:
the ones for whom we care so deeply,
and the ones who have so ably cared for us

Contents

Preface and Acknowledgments

● ●

If I have seen further, it is by standing on ye shoulders of giants.

– Sir Isaac Newton[1]

● ●

This is not your typical book. Originally envisioned as cross between *From Neurons to Neighborhoods*[2] by the Institute of Medicine and Robert D. Putnam's *Our Kids: The American Dream in Crisis,*[3] it is both an approachable summary of developmental science and an unapologetic argument for change. Bringing such a hybrid to fruition has been a "team sport" and a true collaborative effort. Ultimately, it began with the innumerable scientists and investigators over the ages who have applied their skills to better understand the origins of disease and wellness, the mechanisms of human development, and the best ways to translate the latest science into practice and policy. They are the giants who have allowed us to see and expound on the inextricable links between epigenetics, neuroscience, life course theory, the practice of pediatrics, and many of our society's most intractable problems.

But envisioning a book is one thing; actually producing it is quite another. For taking a chance on a hybrid book that was decidedly outside its traditional purview, we are indebted to the American Academy of Pediatrics (AAP). In particular, we are grateful to our developmental editor, Chris Wiberg; the AAP Publishing leadership, including Jeff Mahony and Mark Grimes; Chief Product and Services Officer/SVP, Membership, Marketing, and Publishing Mary Lou White; and the terrific marketing and sales staff, including Kathy Juhl, Sara Hoerdeman, Linda Smessaert, and Elyce Goldstein, led by Marirose Russo and Mark Voigt. We are also thankful for the many reviewers, including Nate Blum, John Duby, Jim Duffee, and Jordan Hutchinson, whose careful attention to detail and clarity has made this book the best it can be.

Finally, as pediatricians, we owe our greatest debt to all of our families. To be sure, our personal families have provided enduring support, encouragement, and patience with us as we have disappeared for days at a time to review the latest research, to reflect on what it might mean, and to obsessively write one draft after another to make a clear and compelling case that the advances in developmental science are transformational. But the families we see in our clinics are the ones that keep us awake each night and inspire us every day. We lose sleep because we know that, despite their parents' best efforts, too many children are not having their most basic biological needs met, and we understand how that sets a questionable foundation for future learning, behavior, and health. Still, we are inspired by these families' unwavering commitment to their children, all too often in the face of tremendous adversity. Their undying resolve to do whatever is best for their children gives us hope that communities can be more caring, families can be more nurturing, and pediatricians can do much more to promote the foundations of lifelong health. But to turn this hope into reality, to expand parents' unquestioned love for their children into a broader appreciation for the power of relational health, and to reframe pediatric care from child-centered to family-centered or even community-centered, there must first be a greater awareness of the recent advances in developmental science. We are most grateful to the entire team for the chance to do just that.

References

1. Newton I. Letter from Sir Isaac Newton to Robert Hooke. Historical Society of Pennsylvania Web site. https://digitallibrary.hsp.org/index.php/Detail/objects/9792. Published February 5, 1675. Accessed December 28, 2017

2. National Research Council, Institute of Medicine. *From Neurons to Neighborhoods: The Science of Early Child Development.* Committee on Integrating the Science of Early Childhood Development. Shonkoff JP, Phillips DA, eds. Washington, DC: National Academy Press; 2000

3. Putnam RD. *Our Kids: The American Dream in Crisis.* New York, NY: Simon & Schuster; 2015

The Pediatric Way

Pediatricians have always been a bit rebellious, but we are rebels with a cause. Our overarching and unwavering cause is to improve the health and well-being of all children. Most physicians strive to be advocates for their patients, but, as pediatricians, we have a long and rich tradition of extending our advocacy beyond our practice walls and into the policies of the broader community. This has always been *the pediatric way:* to translate the latest science into practice and policy to improve the lives of children and their families.

In fact, the very founding of the American Academy of Pediatrics (AAP) as the professional home for physicians focused on the care of children was largely due to a policy rift between the American Medical Association (AMA) Section on Diseases of Children (the professional home for the earliest pediatricians in America) and the AMA House of Delegates.[1] In 1921, Congress passed the Promotion of the Welfare and Hygiene of Maternity and Infancy Act, more commonly known as the Sheppard–Towner Act, which authorized the Children's Bureau to provide matching grants to the states to improve maternal-child health and decrease infant mortality. At the 1922 spring meeting of the AMA, the House of Delegates passed a resolution that condemned the Sheppard–Towner Act on the grounds that it represented governmental intrusion into the practice of medicine and heralded the introduction of socialized medicine.[1] The Section on Diseases of Children, on the other hand, unanimously endorsed this legislation because advances in nutritional science and hygiene made it clear that additional public health measures were needed to improve the lives of children. Incensed that a section would question AMA policy, the House of Delegates subsequently passed a ruling that forbade sections from commenting on AMA policy.

Having silenced internal dissent, the AMA vocally opposed the Sheppard–Towner Act's renewal, even though infant mortality rates fell during its implementation.[2] In 1929, Congress allowed the funding for the act to expire. Left without a voice to support this act and other important public health policies that affected children and their families, early American pediatricians from the AMA Section on Diseases of Children formed the AAP in 1930.[1] By 1934, leaders in this new AAP, including Dr Martha Eliot, helped to draft Title V of the Social Security Act, reviving many of the federal matching programs that were lost when the Sheppard–Towner Act expired.

Hence, from the very beginning, the AAP and American pediatricians recognized the inextricable links between science, medical education, public health, and social policy. At the inaugural AAP Annual Meeting in 1931, the first AAP president, Dr Isaac Abt, stated:

> It will be necessary for the Academy to interest itself in undergraduate education and postgraduate instruction and to exert a regulatory influence over hospitals. As an organization we should assist and lead in public health measures, in social reform, and in hospital and education administration as they affect the welfare of children.[1]

This broad call for pediatricians to support the health and well-being of all children, including those beyond one's individual practice, has become a tradition passed down from one generation of pediatricians to the next. This book is in line with this noble tradition, and it will explore how recent advances in developmental science could transform not only pediatric practice but educational, social, and economic policies as they apply to children and their families.

Grounded in the Science of Development

Ask a group of medical students, "What was the most important lesson that you learned during your pediatrics rotation?" and it is likely that many will respond, "That infants and children are not little adults." But within this patently correct observation lies a subtler, deeper truth: What sets infants and children apart from adults is that infants and children are still under construction. As a consequence, experiences in childhood help to build a strong or weak foundation for future growth.

Similarly, what sets pediatricians apart from other health care professionals is the recognition that their patients are still developing—physically, emotionally, intellectually, and socially. As a consequence, pediatricians must have a fundamental appreciation for the wide array of influences (eg, genetic, nutritional, environmental, social) that affect the unfolding of the developmental process. Pediatricians recognize that current and future child well-being is not just about the child but the developmental milieu: the family, neighborhood, and cultural context in which that development is occurring.

Recently, advances in the basic sciences of development have validated this broader view about the contextual determinants of current and future child health.[3] Life course sciences, including retrospective epidemiological studies of risk[4] and prospective interventional studies,[5] have confirmed what astute pediatricians have known for ages: *What happens in childhood does not necessarily stay in childhood.* At the same time, advances in epigenetics and developmental neuroscience have begun to reveal the underlying mechanisms that allow early childhood experiences to become biologically embedded and to alter life course trajectories for decades to come.[6,7] These advances in the basic sciences of development force us to acknowledge the childhood origins of adult-onset diseases such as hypertension, type 2 diabetes, cancer, and substance abuse, suggesting that many of them are actually adult-*manifest* diseases with their roots in early childhood.

As a consequence of these advances in developmental science, we must reconsider our most basic models of disease and wellness. These advances also challenge us, not only as pediatricians but as parents, educators, policy makers, and citizens, to do a better job of getting genomic function, brain structure, and early relationships right the first time, instead of constantly trying to repair, remediate, and fix seemingly intractable problems down the line. If we can collectively translate this emerging developmental science into practice and policy, we will improve not only current health outcomes but educational, social, and economic outcomes across the life span.[8–10] The pediatric way requires pediatricians to translate this developmental science into practice and policy, but success will require that this pediatric perspective be understood and adopted by more than just the next generation of pediatricians. An understanding of developmental science must become the North Star for all who hope to nurture childhood wellness and promote lifelong health.

About This Book

At its core, *Thinking Developmentally* is about the next generation of pediatricians and the developmental science that will inform their practice and advocacy efforts. But it is also about the next wave of teachers, early childhood professionals, advocates, parents, and others whose efforts could be bolstered by the latest developmental science. Consequently, Part 1 of this book focuses squarely on the latest developmental science. Chapter 1 discusses life course science and the proverbial black box that links *adverse* and *affiliative* experiences in childhood with outcomes decades later. Chapter 2 argues that to peer inside this proverbial black box, we must first ground our understanding of adversity within the body's objective stress *response,* rather than on a wide array of subjective *precipitants* of stress. Chapter 3 explains the burgeoning field of *epigenetics* and how early experiences can be biologically embedded into the way the genome functions. Chapter 4 describes a few principles of developmental neuroscience, the effect of prolonged or *toxic stress responses* on brain development and function, and the concept of *safe, stable, and nurturing relationships* as a powerful antidote to childhood adversity. Chapter 5 ties the entirety of Part 1 together by showing how the advances in developmental science support an ecobiodevelopmental (EBD) model of disease and wellness that forces us all to start *thinking developmentally*. Although we have included essential references to maintain academic rigor, we have attempted to be more approachable than previous discussions of the science to spread these important concepts beyond the hallowed halls of academia. To this end, we have also included a glossary in Appendix A as a handy reference that defines some of the more technical terms, concepts, and abbreviations.

The chapters in Part 2 begin to apply this EBD model to practice and policy. Chapter 6 explores what the most basic, biological needs of children are and what should be done to ensure that those needs are met for all children. The next 4 chapters discuss the implications of the EBD model and the underlying developmental science for parents and caregivers (Chapter 7), communities (Chapter 8), the practice of pediatrics (Chapter 9), and public policy (Chapter 10). We close with an epilogue that reveals our hopes and dreams, not only for this book but for a future that is entirely development informed.

The Tradition Continues

As science has advanced over the last century, pediatricians have worked to translate first the power of adequate nutrition, then public hygiene efforts, later the appropriate use of antibiotics, and still later immunizations into healthier children. As developmental science marches forward, our focus and advocacy strategies must also evolve. But as pediatricians, that's what we do: we translate the latest science into healthy children, nurturing families, and communities that care.

References

1. American Academy of Pediatrics. *Dedicated to the Health of All Children.* Baker JP, Pearson HA, eds. Elk Grove Village, IL: American Academy of Pediatrics; 2005
2. Moehling CM, Thomasson MA. Saving babies: the impact of public education programs on infant mortality. *Demography.* 2014;51(2):367–386
3. National Research Council, Institute of Medicine. *From Neurons to Neighborhoods: The Science of Early Child Development.* Committee on Integrating the Science of Early Childhood Development. Shonkoff JP, Phillips DA, eds. Washington, DC: National Academy Press; 2000

4. Felitti VJ, Anda RF, Nordenberg D, et al. Relationship of childhood abuse and household dysfunction to many of the leading causes of death in adults. The Adverse Childhood Experiences (ACE) Study. *Am J Prev Med.* 1998;14(4):245–258

5. Schweinhart LJ, Montie J, Xiang Z, Barnett WS, Belfield CR, Nores M. *Lifetime Effects: The High/Scope Perry Preschool Study Through Age 40.* Ypsilanti, MI: High/Scope Press; 2005

6. Shonkoff JP, Garner AS; American Academy of Pediatrics Committee on Psychosocial Aspects of Child and Family Health; Committee on Early Childhood, Adoption, and Dependent Care; Section on Developmental and Behavioral Pediatrics. Technical report: the lifelong effects of early childhood adversity and toxic stress. *Pediatrics.* 2012;129(1):e232–e246

7. American Academy of Pediatrics Committee on Psychosocial Aspects of Child and Family Health; Committee on Early Childhood, Adoption, and Dependent Care; Section on Developmental and Behavioral Pediatrics. Policy statement: early childhood adversity, toxic stress, and the role of the pediatrician: translating developmental science into lifelong health. *Pediatrics.* 2012;129(1):e224–e231

8. Shonkoff JP. Building a new biodevelopmental framework to guide the future of early childhood policy. *Child Dev.* 2010;81(1):357–367

9. Shonkoff JP, Boyce WT, McEwen BS. Neuroscience, molecular biology, and the childhood roots of health disparities: building a new framework for health promotion and disease prevention. *JAMA.* 2009;301(21):2252–2259

10. Knudsen EI, Heckman JJ, Cameron JL, Shonkoff JP. Economic, neurobiological, and behavioral perspectives on building America's future workforce. *Proc Natl Acad Sci U S A.* 2006;103(27):10155–10162

Part 1: Advances in Developmental Science

Chapter 1

Life Course Science and the Proverbial Black Box

As pediatricians, parents, teachers, and citizens, what do we wish for the children in our lives? For them to be healthy? Happy? Productive? Ultimately, we want our children to thrive, not only in childhood but across their life span. We want them to fulfill their potential, to make a difference in the world, and to positively influence generations to come. As such, we tend to measure success not in the short term but over the life course. We may worry about recurrent ear infections in a young girl because they may affect her hearing as she gets older. We might worry about a boy's early struggles in elementary school because they may diminish his ability to graduate high school or college or to get a good-paying job. We intuitively understand that what happens in childhood may not stay in childhood.

But we also understand that what happens in early childhood is not necessarily destiny. We all know examples of healthy, happy, and productive adults who overcame tremendous adversity as children, just as we know teenagers and adults who benefitted from every possible resource as children but nevertheless fared poorly over the years. The link between childhood experiences and adult outcomes is strong, but it is not perfect, and this ambiguity poses important questions: What adversities in childhood alter life course trajectories for the worse? What are the essential ingredients of *good-enough parenting* (to be discussed more in Chapter 7) that alter life course trajectories for the better? Where can differences be made in what we do as parents, pediatricians, teachers, and neighbors?

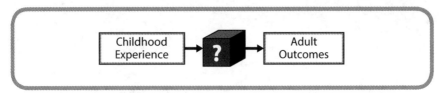

Figure 1-1. Defining the proverbial black box that links experiences in childhood with outcomes decades later. To advance health, educational, and economic outcomes across the life span, we need to peer inside this black box and better understand the biological mechanisms underlying these well-established associations.

In this chapter, we will briefly review the associations between experiences in childhood and outcomes in health, behavior, and economic productivity decades later. We conceptualize this process as a black box. We know what goes into the box: early childhood experiences, both *adverse* (negative, harmful, isolating) and *affiliative* (positive, affirming, inclusive). We also know what comes out of the box: childhood, adolescent, and adult outcomes. However, what goes on *inside* the box—the biological mechanisms underlying these strong but imperfect associations—has, until recently, remained poorly understood (Figure 1-1). Only by peering inside this black box and understanding the biological mechanisms at play will we be able to ensure a good beginning and set a steady course toward a good end. But here we will begin by looking at those pivotal inputs as well as the outputs of utmost concern.

Life Course Science

Advances in life course sciences, like epidemiology and intervention science, are confirming that the link between childhood experiences and adult outcomes is quite strong. For example, the landmark Adverse Childhood Experiences (ACE) Study[1,2] asked more than 17,000 middle-class, middle-aged Americans if they had experienced any of the following 10 categories of adversity (Table 1-1) prior to their 18th birthday: emotional (psychological) abuse, physical abuse, sexual abuse, mother treated violently (ie, witnessing intimate partner violence), household substance abuse, household mental illness, parental separation or divorce, an incarcerated household member, emotional neglect, and physical neglect. The lead researchers of the ACE Study, Drs Vincent Felitti and Robert Anda, were astonished to see just how prevalent these ACEs were, with more than one-quarter of the participants reporting physical abuse and household substance abuse prior to their adulthood. Moreover, sexual abuse, parental separation or divorce, and household

Table 1-1. Adverse Childhood Experiences Are Not Rare

	Women (n = 9,367)	Men (n = 7,970)	Total (N = 17,337)
Abuse			
• Emotional	13.1	7.6	10.6
• Physical	27.0	29.9	28.3
• Sexual	24.7	16.0	20.7
Household dysfunction			
• Mother treated violently	13.7	11.5	12.7
• Household substance abuse	29.5	23.8	26.9
• Household mental illness	23.3	14.8	19.4
• Parental separation or divorce	24.5	21.8	23.3
• Incarcerated household member	5.2	4.1	4.7
Neglect[a]			
• Emotional	16.7	12.4	14.8
• Physical	9.2	10.7	9.9

[a] Wave 2 data only (n = 8,667).

Data from www.cdc.gov/violenceprevention/acestudy.

The Adverse Childhood Experiences (ACE) Study asked more than 17,000 middle-class adults to recall if they had experienced any of the 10 listed adversities prior to their 18th birthday. The percentage of participants who experienced each category of ACE is given for women and men. To determine an individual's ACE score, 1 point was given for each type of ACE recalled (for a maximum score of 10). Only 36% of the participants had an ACE score of 0, and 1 in 8 had an ACE score of 4 or more.

From Garner AS. Home visiting and the biology of toxic stress: opportunities to address early childhood adversity. *Pediatrics.* 2013;132(Suppl 2):S65–S73.

mental illness were each reported by about 1 in 5 participants during their first 18 years of life.

When these data were first published in 1998, they were met with a great deal of skepticism because the original ACE Study was conducted on a population (primarily white and well educated) that might be expected to have experienced minimal adversity in childhood.[1] However, subsequent studies have confirmed that ACEs are indeed quite common, and they are even more common in underprivileged populations, like those living in poverty[3] or subjected to incarceration.[4]

To quantify this childhood adversity, the authors developed an ACE score encompassing 10 different categories of adversity. Participants were given 1 point for each category they had experienced during their childhood. Here again, the prevalence of high ACE scores was shocking, with about two-thirds (64%) having an ACE score of 1 or higher, and 1 in 8 (12.5%) having an ACE score of 4 or higher.[1] As disturbing as these numbers are, it is important to remember that the ACE score is actually a relatively insensitive measure of adversity for several reasons. First, because the original ACE Study was retrospective (most participants were in their 50s and were asked about experiences that had happened prior to their 18th birthday), issues with recall may lower the ACE score, as people may repress or try to forget upsetting experiences.[5] Second, the ACE score does not account for frequency or repetition. Whether a participant was sexually abused one time or every day for years, the participant received only 1 ACE point. Finally, redundancy is possible within the 10 categories: a participant may have had an alcoholic father and a mother who was a chronic marijuana user, but that participant would have received only 1 ACE point for the category of household substance abuse. These limitations suggest that, if anything, ACE scores underestimate the true prevalence of childhood adversity.

Despite these limitations, Felitti, Anda, and colleagues were able to demonstrate graded, dose-dependent, and statistically significant relationships between ACE scores and a wide array of outcomes (Box 1-1).[1,2] These outcomes included not only common diseases (eg, cancer, ischemic heart disease, chronic lung disease, liver disease) but measures of sexual health (eg, early intercourse, teen pregnancy, sexually transmitted infections, sexual dissatisfaction), mental health (eg, anxiety, depression, hallucinations, panic reactions [attacks], poor anger control), and general or social functioning (eg, relationship problems, difficulty at work, high perceived stress). The list of outcomes associated with ACEs is almost overwhelming, but this also underscores a tremendous potential for benefit. If we are able to understand the biological mechanisms underlying these associations, we are in a better position to address and, hopefully, prevent a wide array of seemingly intractable outcomes.

The opportunities for prevention are even more promising when one considers that adverse experiences in childhood were associated, in adulthood, with what we will call *the Big 5:* smoking, alcoholism, obesity, promiscuity,

Box 1-1. Adverse Childhood Experiences Are Associated With Numerous Measures of Poor Health

I. Social Functioning
a. High Perceived Stress
b. Relationship Problems
c. Married to an Alcoholic
d. Difficulty With Job
II. Mental Health
a. Anxiety
b. Depression
c. Poor Anger Control
d. Panic Reactions
e. Sleep Disturbances
f. Memory Disturbances
g. Hallucinations
III. Sexual Health
a. Age of First Intercourse
b. Unintended Pregnancy
c. Teen Pregnancy
d. Teen Paternity
e. Fetal Death
f. Sexual Dissatisfaction
IV. Risk Factors for Common Diseases
a. Obesity
b. Promiscuity
c. Alcoholism
d. Smoking
e. Illicit Drugs
f. IV Drugs
g. High Perceived Risk of HIV
h. Multiple Somatic Symptoms
V. Prevalent Diseases
a. Ischemic Heart Disease
b. Chronic Lung Disease
c. Liver Disease
d. Cancer
e. Skeletal Fractures
f. Sexual Transmitted Infections

Abbreviations: ACE, Adverse Childhood Experiences; HIV, human immunodeficiency virus; IV, intravenous.

All these adolescent and adult outcomes are associated with ACE scores in a dose-dependent and statistically significant manner. The higher the ACE score, the higher the risk for these measures of poor health. Note that the Big 5 (overeating [a proxy for obesity], sex, alcohol, smoking, and substance abuse) are behaviors that transiently turn off stress and that they, in turn, are associated with most of the other outcomes associated with childhood adversity. For example, overeating is associated with heart disease, promiscuity is associated with sexual health dysfunction, alcoholism is associated with liver disease and social difficulties, smoking is associated with chronic lung disease, and substance abuse is associated with social difficulties and mental health conditions.

Adapted from Centers for Disease Control and Prevention. Adverse childhood experiences (ACEs). www.cdc.gov/violenceprevention/acestudy. Updated April 1, 2016. Accessed February 27, 2018.

From Garner AS. Home visiting and the biology of toxic stress: opportunities to address early childhood adversity. *Pediatrics.* 2013;132(Suppl 2):S65–S73.

and substance abuse. Each of these is a well-established risk factor for disease. In fact, many of the other outcomes associated with ACEs are known to be related to these Big 5. For example, if you are obese, that increases your risks for hypertension, diabetes, and heart disease. If you are alcoholic, that increases your risk of having liver disease and other forms of cancer. If you are a smoker, that increases your risk of chronic lung disease and many types of cancer. If you are promiscuous, that increases your risk of sexually transmitted infections (including HIV and hepatitis C), early parenting, and poor sexual health. Finally, substance abuse and alcoholism are associated with mental health conditions and other measures of poor general or social functioning.

Behavioral Allostasis

What is driving the relationship between ACE scores and the Big 5? Physiologists would point out that the Big 5 are all examples of *behavioral allostasis*.[6-8] The term *allostasis* refers to the active process that the body uses to get back to baseline after being altered by the environment. For example, if the body's core temperature begins to rise, allostasis is manifest on the redirection of blood flow to the skin to dissipate heat. Similarly, behavioral allostasis refers to behaviors that return the body's functioning back to baseline. In the case of the Big 5 (tobacco, alcohol, overeating [as a proxy for obesity], sex, and substance abuse), they all provide an opportunity to transiently turn off stress, allowing us to relax, if only for a moment. While it might seem intuitive that significant adversity is associated with the Big 5 and other risky behaviors (eg, compulsive gambling[9]) that provide a rush of positive feelings or transiently turn off stress, it may be surprising to consider that these stress-modulating behaviors are occurring decades after the original childhood adversity. Even more surprising is the fact that ACEs increase the risk of disease—ischemic heart disease, for example— even after controlling for the Big 5 and other traditional risk factors for disease.[10] This means that someone who has suffered significant childhood adversity is at a higher risk of ischemic heart disease even if he or she does not have any of the associated behavioral risk factors. This raises an intriguing question: Are ACEs getting under the skin, becoming biologically embedded and driving health, behavior, and economic outcomes over the entire life course? We will return to this question and address it more thoroughly in chapters 3 and 4.

Of course, the adversities examined in the ACE Study are not the only ones associated with poor adult outcomes. Other known risk factors for poor outcomes later in life include growing up in poverty, being bullied, witnessing violence, experiencing other forms of parental dysfunction (eg, harsh or belittling parents), or living in a violent neighborhood. While it seems intuitive that *catastrophic* adversities (eg, physical abuse, sexual abuse, witnessing violence) might be associated with poor outcomes, the retrospective ACE Study and several smaller prospective studies have demonstrated that *chronic* adversities (eg, maternal depression, poverty, emotional neglect) are also associated with poor outcomes.[11-14] When we explore what is going on inside the black box, we must consider catastrophic and chronic sources of adversity (Figure 1-2).[15]

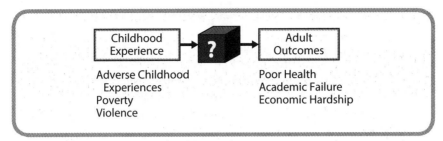

Figure 1-2. Adverse experiences, both catastrophic (eg, violence) and chronic (eg, poverty), are associated with outcomes like poor health, academic failure, and economic hardship later in life. To break this association and improve outcomes, we need to understand the biological mechanisms at play inside the black box.

The good news is that childhood experiences appear to cut both ways. Although adversities are associated with poor outcomes, sources of enrichment during childhood are associated with improved outcomes in behavior, learning, and health (Figure 1-3). For example, *affiliative* childhood experiences, like engaged, attentive caregivers; access to health care; quality early education services; and even ample opportunities to play, have been associated with lifelong outcomes such as better health,[16] higher academic achievement, more employment, fewer divorces, less depression, and lower incarceration rates.[17-19]

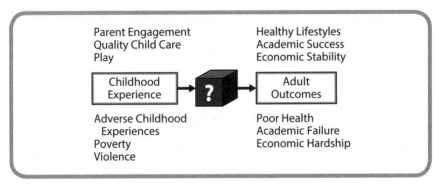

Figure 1-3. Affiliative childhood experiences, like parental engagement, quality child care, and opportunities to play, are associated with outcomes like healthy lifestyles, academic success, and economic stability later in life. An understanding of the biological mechanisms working inside the box is absolutely necessary for preventing the negative outcomes associated with adverse childhood experiences, promoting the positive outcomes associated with affiliative childhood experiences, and addressing many of society's most intractable problems, like disparities in health, education, and economic productivity.

Summary

Early childhood experiences, both affiliative and adverse, are strongly associated with important outcomes later in life. The challenge now is to begin looking into this black box to understand the biological mechanisms underlying these well-established associations and to translate this knowledge into practices and policies that will address and perhaps even prevent many of our society's most intractable problems. Understanding the biological mechanisms within the black box is requisite knowledge for pediatricians, parents, teachers, advocates, policy makers, and all others interested in fostering healthy children, resilient teens, and the next generation of productive, civic-minded adults.

References

1. Felitti VJ, Anda RF, Nordenberg D, et al. Relationship of childhood abuse and household dysfunction to many of the leading causes of death in adults. The Adverse Childhood Experiences (ACE) Study. *Am J Prev Med.* 1998;14(4):245–258
2. Anda RF, Felitti VJ, Bremner JD, et al. The enduring effects of abuse and related adverse experiences in childhood. A convergence of evidence from neurobiology and epidemiology. *Eur Arch Psychiatry Clin Neurosci.* 2006;256(3):174–186
3. Bucci M, Marques SS, Oh D, Harris NB. Toxic stress in children and adolescents. *Adv Pediatr.* 2016;63(1):403–428
4. Naramore R, Bright MA, Epps N, Hardt NS. Youth arrested for trading sex have the highest rates of childhood adversity: a statewide study of juvenile offenders. *Sex Abuse.* 2017;29(4):396–410
5. Axmacher N, Do Lam AT, Kessler H, Fell J. Natural memory beyond the storage model: repression, trauma, and the construction of a personal past. *Front Hum Neurosci.* 2010;4:211
6. Karatsoreos IN, McEwen BS. Psychobiological allostasis: resistance, resilience and vulnerability. *Trends Cogn Sci.* 2011;15(12):576–584
7. McEwen BS. Physiology and neurobiology of stress and adaptation: central role of the brain. *Physiol Rev.* 2007;87(3):873–904
8. McEwen BS, Wingfield JC. The concept of allostasis in biology and biomedicine. *Horm Behav.* 2003;43(1):2–15
9. Scherrer JF, Xian H, Kapp JM, et al. Association between exposure to childhood and lifetime traumatic events and lifetime pathological gambling in a twin cohort. *J Nerv Ment Dis.* 2007;195(1):72–78
10. Dong M, Giles WH, Felitti VJ, et al. Insights into causal pathways for ischemic heart disease: Adverse Childhood Experiences Study. *Circulation.* 2004;110(13):1761–1766
11. Flaherty EG, Thompson R, Litrownik AJ, et al. Effect of early childhood adversity on child health. *Arch Pediatr Adolesc Med.* 2006;160(12):1232–1238
12. Koenen KC, Moffitt TE, Poulton R, Martin J, Caspi A. Early childhood factors associated with the development of post-traumatic stress disorder: results from a longitudinal birth cohort. *Psychol Med.* 2007;37(2):181–192
13. Danese A, Moffitt TE, Harrington H, et al. Adverse childhood experiences and adult risk factors for age-related disease: depression, inflammation, and clustering of metabolic risk markers. *Arch Pediatr Adolesc Med.* 2009;163(12):1135–1143

14. Flaherty EG, Thompson R, Litrownik AJ, et al. Adverse childhood exposures and reported child health at age 12. *Acad Pediatr.* 2009;9(3):150–156
15. Odgers CL, Jaffee SR. Routine versus catastrophic influences on the developing child. *Annu Rev Public Health.* 2013;34:29–48
16. Campbell F, Conti G, Heckman JJ, et al. Early childhood investments substantially boost adult health. *Science.* 2014;343(6178):1478–1485
17. Schweinhart LJ, Montie J, Xiang Z, Barnett WS, Belfield CR, Nores M. *Lifetime Effects: The High/Scope Perry Preschool Study Through Age 40.* Ypsilanti, MI: High/Scope Press; 2005
18. McLaughlin AE, Campbell FA, Pungello EP, Skinner M. Depressive symptoms in young adults: the influences of the early home environment and early educational child care. *Child Dev.* 2007;78(3):746–756
19. Walker SP, Chang SM, Vera-Hernández M, Grantham-McGregor S. Early childhood stimulation benefits adult competence and reduces violent behavior. *Pediatrics.* 2011;127(5):849–857

Chapter 2

Defining Adversity and Toxic Stress

· ·

It is your reaction to adversity, not the adversity itself,
that determines how your life's story will develop.

– *Dieter Uchtdorf*

· ·

The Adverse Childhood Experiences (ACE) Study and other recent advances in life course science discussed in Chapter 1 highlight the need to think longitudinally across the life span, to peer inside the black box, and to understand the biology underlying well-established associations between experiences in childhood and outcomes decades later. A more sophisticated understanding of how adverse and affiliative experiences in childhood alter life course trajectories has tremendous implications for practice and policy. But an acknowledgment that early experiences are biologically embedded would also force us to reconsider the childhood origins of lifelong disease and wellness. A broader discussion of various models of disease and wellness appears in Chapter 5, but few models to date have incorporated the recent advances in life course and developmental science. Therefore, one of the objectives of this book is to fashion a model of disease and wellness that is squarely grounded in this potentially transformative developmental science.

The life course science discussed in Chapter 1 is summarized in a different manner in Figure 2-1. The salient features of the early childhood ecology, positive and negative, are strongly associated with developmental outcomes, not only in childhood and adolescence but decades later. Salient features of the ecology include not only the climate and physical or built environment but also the nutritional, cultural, and social-emotional milieu in which children are raised. As discussed in Chapter 1, the developmental outcomes of utmost interest are not limited to health but include behaviors and lifestyles, academic success, and economic productivity. The dashed arrow

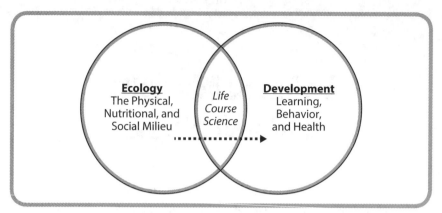

Figure 2-1. The early childhood ecology includes the physical, nutritional, and social environment and is strongly associated (dashed line) with lifelong developmental outcomes in learning, behavior, and health.

in Figure 2-1 indicates that, although the ecology is strongly associated with these lifelong developmental outcomes, these links may or may not be causal. To peer inside the black box and to understand the biological mechanisms underlying these associations, we must first find a way to measure or quantify the ecology. In the case of ACEs, we need to find a way to measure or quantify adversity and stress.

The Perception of Adversity Is Subjective, but the Reaction Is Not

The problem with adversity and stress is that they are both extremely subjective, making them hard to measure or quantify. One person's exciting opportunity is an overwhelming challenge to another. One child hears a dog bark and thinks, "Puppy—let's play," whereas another is terrified by the very same sound. Differences in the way individuals perceive a given threat or adversity certainly play a pivotal role in determining which individuals respond to that threat or adversity in a resilient versus maladaptive manner, but there are innumerable factors at play when it comes to how a given threat or adversity is perceived. Previous experiences, cultural norms, family traditions, and biological predilections all color how we see the world, influencing what we identify as a threat and what we perceive as an adversity. This wide degree of individual variability in the perception of stress suggests that the way to measure or define adversity rests not in the various precipitants of stress or in the adversities themselves but in the reaction—the type of biological responses they trigger. That said, many interventions to assist those who are already traumatized focus on changing the way the threat or adversity is perceived or understood.[1,2]

The Basics of the Body's Stress Response
Amygdala

Although the perception of a threat is highly variable, once a potential threat is perceived, the mechanics of the body's stress response are more uniform. Threat perception first activates the amygdala, a heterogeneous collection of nuclei considered to be a major center of emotional processing and response within the brain.[3–5] The amygdala, in turn, activates several known pathways that eventually lead to 4 major behavioral responses to a threat: *freeze, flight, fight,* or *affiliate* (Figure 2-2). Most of this chapter will focus on the mechanics

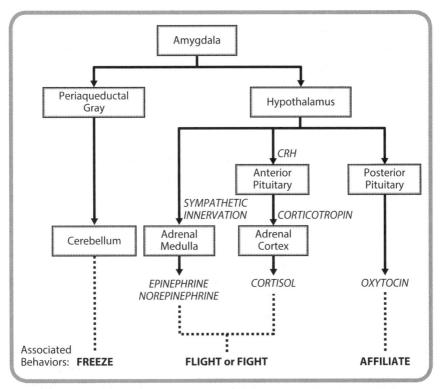

Figure 2-2. The amygdala's integral role in the 4 major behavioral responses to a threat. A *freeze* response includes amygdala activation of the periaqueductal gray and, in turn, the cerebellum. Although not shown in this figure, freezing also involves amygdala activation of the parasympathetic nervous system (the vagal nerve via the hypothalamus) and a slowing of the heart rate. A freeze response is thought to represent an active brake on a motor system that is preparing for imminent flight or fight. A *flight or fight* response includes amygdala activation of the adrenal medulla and cortex through the sympathetic nervous system and the anterior pituitary (via the hypothalamus). Mediators like epinephrine, norepinephrine, and cortisol assist the body in actually fleeing or fighting. Finally, an *affiliate* response includes amygdala activation of the hypothalamus and the release of oxytocin from the posterior pituitary. Although not shown in this figure, oxytocin provides a negative feedback loop by inhibiting activation of the amygdala and the use of the other behavioral responses.[6] (Abbreviation: CRH, corticotropin-releasing hormone.)

underlying the flight or fight response because the pathways underlying these responses are well defined. More importantly, the mediators of the flight or fight response (eg, cortisol) are known to have long-lasting effects on the genome, brain, and immune system. But here it is worth noting that there are 2 other behavioral responses to perceived threats (freeze and affiliate) that are well established in animal models and are emerging areas of human research.

Freeze

In animal models and humans, a freeze response involves the tonic activation of muscle groups, includes a relative slowing of the heart rate, is thought to represent a flight or fight response that is temporarily put on hold, and involves the amygdala's activation of the periaqueductal gray.[7] Anecdotally, we are all familiar with the "deer in the headlights" response or the concept of being paralyzed by fear, and this amygdala-activated pathway through the periaqueductal gray likely plays a major role in these responses to a perceived threat.

Affiliate

The behavioral response to affiliate in response to a threat, also known as "tend and befriend,"[8] is seen in many mammalian species.[9–11] The peptide hormone oxytocin is thought to play a major role in mediating this response. When stress and anxiety activate the amygdala, it, in turn, signals the hypothalamus to increase oxytocin into the peripheral bloodstream (via the posterior pituitary) and other centers within the brain. Oxytocin is known to promote pro-social perceptions, thoughts, and behaviors. For example, it is known to improve the recognition of social cues, to increase trust and positive communications, and to promote a mother's bonding with her child.[6] Most importantly, oxytocin goes up in response to positive social interactions (eg, affectionate physical contact), and it provides a negative feedback loop to the amygdala, thereby decreasing subjective stress and anxiety.[6] Although a full discussion of the complex but intriguing role of oxytocin in pro-social behaviors is beyond the scope of this book,[6,9] it is worth noting here that oxytocin is likely to play an important role in the way that safe, stable, and nurturing relationships buffer childhood adversity. If future research is able to discern the integrative processes governing which of the 4 behavioral responses is selected in response to a threat, it could allow for better interventions to assist individuals who get locked into the same recurring patterns in response to adversity or threats (eg, freeze or fight rather than affiliate).[12]

Flight or Fight: The Sympatho-adrenomedullary Pathway

The amygdala also prepares the body for flight and fight behaviors through 2 distinct hypothalamic pathways: the sympatho-adrenomedullary (SAM) pathway and the hypothalamic-pituitary-adrenal (HPA) axis (Figure 2-3). In the SAM pathway, the neurons of the hypothalamospinal tract activate the sympathetic nervous system, which, in turn, stimulates the adrenal medulla to release epinephrine and norepinephrine. These hormones rapidly induce biological changes, like elevations in heart rate, blood pressure, and blood glucose levels. In life-threatening situations, these rapid changes prepare the body

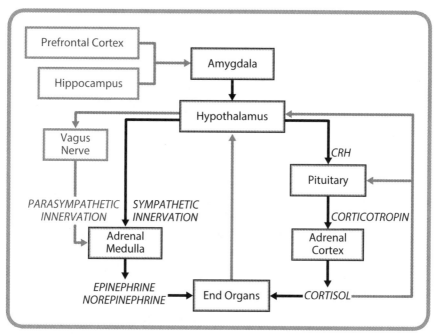

Figure 2-3. The basic elements and regulation of the flight or fight response system. Once threats are perceived by the amygdala, it signals the hypothalamus to activate 2 complementary pathways. In the hypothalamic-pituitary-adrenal axis, the release of corticotropin-releasing hormone (CRH) by the hypothalamus stimulates the pituitary to release corticotropin. In the adrenal cortex, corticotropin stimulates the release of cortisol into the bloodstream. In the sympatho-adrenomedullary pathway, the hypothalamus activates the sympathetic nervous system, and sympathetic innervation of the adrenal medulla stimulates the release of epinephrine and norepinephrine into the bloodstream. Important regulators of the stress response system are shown in gray. The prefrontal cortex and the hippocampus inhibit the activity of the amygdala. Parasympathetic innervation of the adrenal medulla via the vagus nerve inhibits the release of epinephrine and norepinephrine. Cortisol downregulates its own production via negative feedback loops to the hypothalamus and pituitary. Finally, end-organ functions (eg, blood pressure, blood glucose levels) are also monitored and regulated by the hypothalamus.

for flight or fight. In the short term, such biological changes might increase the probability of survival from a singular threat, but if they are sustained (eg, prolonged elevations in blood pressure or glucose levels), they may also prove to be damaging.[13-17] Hence, the regulation and time course of the physiologic stress response are absolutely pivotal. Too little of a stress response, and you might become dinner for a predator. But if the stress response is sustained (once the predator is gone, or if you perceive that a predator is always nearby), you may die early of cardiovascular disease or diabetes.[18-24]

Flight or Fight: The Hypothalamic-pituitary-adrenal Axis

In the HPA axis, the paraventricular nucleus of the hypothalamus secretes corticotropin-releasing hormone, which stimulates the release of corticotropin from the anterior lobe of the pituitary. Corticotropin stimulates the synthesis and release of cortisol from the adrenal gland, and cortisol then acts on glucocorticoid receptors throughout the body. Although the body's response to cortisol (minutes to hours) is slower than the response to epinephrine (seconds), cortisol also induces changes in physiologic processes that might be considered adaptive in a life-threatening situation, including increases in blood glucose levels (energy for the muscles), dampening the immune response (no fevers in the midst of a fight), and altering memory function (no reminiscing while on the run). In sum, cortisol and the HPA axis also support the body's flight or fight response, but over a slower time course. In addition, excessive exposure to cortisol induces downstream biological changes in gene expression (see Chapter 3) and brain connectivity (see Chapter 4) that may persist for a long time (hours, days, even years) after the initial threat is gone.

Regulating the Body's Stress Response

Because the mediators of the body's stress response (eg, cortisol, epinephrine, norepinephrine) can be lifesaving or life-threatening depending on their magnitude and time course, their release is highly regulated (see Figure 2-3). This regulation begins in the brain as the prefrontal cortex and hippocampus inhibit the activation of the amygdala. (This regulation at the level of the amygdala will be discussed more in Chapter 4.) In the case of the SAM pathway, the vagal nerve, a branch of the parasympathetic nervous system, helps to turn off the secretion of the hormones from the adrenal medulla. This has led some researchers to consider ways to promote vagal function as a means of countering chronic stress.[9] In the case of the HPA axis, glucocorticoid receptors in the hypothalamus and pituitary form a negative feedback loop that allows cortisol to downregulate its own production. When threats are rare and brief, the body's stress response system works like a well-oiled machine, upregulating in response to a perceived threat and downregulating when the threat has passed. When threats are frequent or sustained, the body's stress response system adapts by initially becoming more active, but over time it may eventually become "exhausted" and dysregulated.[25–31]

Rather than directly measuring the levels of these important mediators (eg, cortisol, epinephrine, norepinephrine), many investigations of the body's stress response look at the consequences these mediators have for bodily functions like blood pressure, heart rate, and respiratory patterns. Measuring these mediators directly can be difficult because, among other reasons, cortisol levels have a diurnal cycle, and drawing blood or taking a measurement can be an artificial stressor that affects the result. Nonetheless, these known, objective *responses* to stress and adversity are quantified more easily than a wide array of potential and subjective *precipitants* of stress.

A Taxonomy of Stress Responses

Jack Shonkoff and his colleagues on the National Scientific Council on the Developing Child have suggested a taxonomy of stress[32] based on the objective, quantifiable responses to adversity: *positive stress, tolerable stress,* and *toxic stress* (Table 2-1).

Positive Stress

Positive stress responses are brief, mild in intensity, and relatively infrequent.[33,34] They are often triggered by the minor adversities experienced by children every day. Examples of such minor adversities include the inability of a 15-month-old to express herself, a toddler who stumbles while he is learning to walk, a young child who must leave her mother on the first day of kindergarten, and a middle schooler who is intimidated by the prospect of tackling that big, month-long project. The biological responses to these adversities are typically brief and mild, and the body's stress response system returns to baseline relatively quickly due to the presence of safe, stable, and nurturing relationships. Such relationships turn off the stress response by responding to nonverbal cues, offering consolation, providing reassurance, and dividing an overwhelming challenge into smaller, more manageable pieces. In the presence of safe, stable, and nurturing relationships, minor adversities actually build motivation and lead to competence and confidence. It is important to note that positive stress is not the absence of stress but the ability to cope with the adversity in an adaptive and healthy manner. As parents, teachers, and pediatricians, our objective is not to put our children in a stress-free bubble but to teach them the skills they need to adapt to any adversity in a healthy way.

Table 2-1. A Taxonomy of Stress

Physiologic Stress in Childhood			
Stress Response	Positive	Tolerable	Toxic
Duration	Brief	Sustained	Sustained
Severity	Mild/ moderate	Moderate/ severe	Severe
Social-Emotional Buffering (Safe, Stable, and Nurturing Relationships)	Sufficient	Sufficient	Insufficient
Long-term Effect on Stress Response System	Return to baseline	Return to baseline	Changes to baseline

Biological Alterations	
• Epigenetic modifications. • Changes in brain structure and function. • Behavioral allostasis/ attempts to cope.	• All these alterations may prove to be maladaptive in other contexts.

Modified from American Academy of Pediatrics. *Bright Futures: Guidelines for Health Supervision of Infants, Children, and Adolescents.* Hagan JF, Shaw JS, Duncan PM, eds. 4th ed. Elk Grove Village, IL: American Academy of Pediatrics; 2017.

Tolerable Stress

Tolerable stress responses are not as brief, are more intense, or may occur more frequently than positive stress responses.[33,34] Examples of adversities that might precipitate tolerable stress responses include the death of a parent, moving away from friends, or frequent social dramas that fall just short of bullying. These adversities trigger stress responses that have the potential to induce long-lasting biological changes but fail to do so in the presence of the safe, stable, and nurturing relationships that buffer adversity by turning off the body's stress response. However, unlike positive stress responses, tolerable stress responses may not build motivation or lead to competence and confidence.

Toxic Stress

Toxic stress responses are long-lasting, severe in intensity, or frequent.[33,34] The ACEs discussed in Chapter 1 are examples of events that might trigger a toxic stress response, because even the strong social-emotional buffering provided by safe, stable, and nurturing relationships may be insufficient to completely turn off the body's stress response. As a consequence of a prolonged exposure to the mediators of the physiologic stress response (eg, cortisol, epinephrine, norepinephrine), potentially permanent biological changes take place through at least 2 known mechanisms: epigenetics and developmental neuroscience. These biologically related but conceptually distinct mechanisms will be discussed in more detail in chapters 3 and 4, respectively. Understanding these mechanisms is paramount because they allow early childhood experiences to become biologically embedded and to influence behavior, learning, and health decades later.

Summary

The way to measure or define adversity rests not in the varied and subjective precipitants of stress but in the type of objective, biological responses they trigger. Positive stress responses are brief and build competence and confidence in the face of future adversity. But prolonged exposure to the mediators of the body's stress response, especially in the absence of safe, stable, and nurturing relationships, can drive potentially permanent biological changes in genomic function and brain architecture that, while adaptive and survival-promoting in the short term, may ultimately prove maladaptive or toxic over time.

References

1. van der Kolk BA. The neurobiology of childhood trauma and abuse. *Child Adolesc Psychiatr Clin N Am.* 2003;12(2):293–317
2. Cisler JM, Sigel BA, Kramer TL, et al. Amygdala response predicts trajectory of symptom reduction during trauma-focused cognitive-behavioral therapy among adolescent girls with PTSD. *J Psychiatr Res.* 2015;71:33–40
3. Tottenham N, Sheridan MA. A review of adversity, the amygdala and the hippocampus: a consideration of developmental timing. *Front Hum Neurosci.* 2009;3:68
4. Kim P, Evans GW, Angstadt M, et al. Effects of childhood poverty and chronic stress on emotion regulatory brain function in adulthood. *Proc Natl Acad Sci U S A.* 2013;110(46):18442–18447
5. McEwen BS, Gianaros PJ. Central role of the brain in stress and adaptation: links to socioeconomic status, health, and disease. *Ann N Y Acad Sci.* 2010;1186:190–222
6. Meyer-Lindenberg A, Domes G, Kirsch P, Heinrichs M. Oxytocin and vasopressin in the human brain: social neuropeptides for translational medicine. *Nat Rev Neurosci.* 2011;12(9):524–538

7. Roelofs K. Freeze for action: neurobiological mechanisms in animal and human freezing. *Philos Trans R Soc Lond B Biol Sci.* 2017;372(1718):20160206
8. Taylor SE, Klein LC, Lewis BP, Gruenewald TL, Gurung RA, Updegraff JA. Biobehavioral responses to stress in females: tend-and-befriend, not fight-or-flight. *Psychol Rev.* 2000;107(3):411–429
9. Porges SW. *The Polyvagal Theory: Neurophysiological Foundations of Emotions, Attachment, Communication, and Self-Regulation.* New York, NY: W. W. Norton and Co; 2011
10. Porges SW. The polyvagal theory: phylogenetic contributions to social behavior. *Physiol Behav.* 2003;79(3):503–513
11. Porges SW. Social engagement and attachment: a phylogenetic perspective. *Ann N Y Acad Sci.* 2003;1008:31–47
12. Kozlowska K, Walker P, McLean L, Carrive P. Fear and the defense cascade: clinical implications and management. *Harv Rev Psychiatry.* 2015;23(4):263–287
13. Juster RP, Bizik G, Picard M, et al. A transdisciplinary perspective of chronic stress in relation to psychopathology throughout life span development. *Dev Psychopathol.* 2011;23(3):725–776
14. McEwen BS, Gianaros PJ. Stress- and allostasis-induced brain plasticity. *Annu Rev Med.* 2011;62:431–445
15. Juster RP, McEwen BS, Lupien SJ. Allostatic load biomarkers of chronic stress and impact on health and cognition. *Neurosci Biobehav Rev.* 2010;35(1):2–16
16. McEwen BS. Central effects of stress hormones in health and disease: understanding the protective and damaging effects of stress and stress mediators. *Eur J Pharmacol.* 2008;583(2-3):174–185
17. McEwen BS. Protective and damaging effects of stress mediators: central role of the brain. *Dialogues Clin Neurosci.* 2006;8(4):367–381
18. Duru OK, Harawa NT, Kermah D, Norris KC. Allostatic load burden and racial disparities in mortality. *J Natl Med Assoc.* 2012;104(1-2):89–95
19. Dong M, Giles WH, Felitti VJ, et al. Insights into causal pathways for ischemic heart disease: adverse childhood experiences study. *Circulation.* 2004;110(13):1761–1766
20. McEwen BS, Wingfield JC. The concept of allostasis in biology and biomedicine. *Horm Behav.* 2003;43(1):2–15
21. Anda RF, Felitti VJ, Bremner JD, et al. The enduring effects of abuse and related adverse experiences in childhood. A convergence of evidence from neurobiology and epidemiology. *Eur Arch Psychiatry Clin Neurosci.* 2006;256(3):174–186
22. Felitti VJ, Anda RF, Nordenberg D, et al. Relationship of childhood abuse and household dysfunction to many of the leading causes of death in adults. The Adverse Childhood Experiences (ACE) Study. *Am J Prev Med.* 1998;14(4):245–258
23. Brown DW, Anda RF, Tiemeier H, et al. Adverse childhood experiences and the risk of premature mortality. *Am J Prev Med.* 2009;37(5):389–396
24. Anda RF, Dong M, Brown DW, et al. The relationship of adverse childhood experiences to a history of premature death of family members. *BMC Public Health.* 2009;9:106
25. Pagliaccio D, Luby JL, Bogdan R, et al. Stress-system genes and life stress predict cortisol levels and amygdala and hippocampal volume in children. *Neuropsychopharmacology.* 2014;39(5):1245–1253
26. Power C, Thomas C, Li L, Hertzman C. Childhood psychosocial adversity and adult cortisol patterns. *Br J Psychiatry.* 2012;201(3):199–206
27. Badanes LS, Watamura SE, Hankin BL. Hypocortisolism as a potential marker of allostatic load in children: associations with family risk and internalizing disorders. *Dev Psychopathol.* 2011;23(3):881–896

28. Bush NR, Obradović J, Adler N, Boyce WT. Kindergarten stressors and cumulative adrenocortical activation: the "first straws" of allostatic load? *Dev Psychopathol.* 2011;23(4):1089–1106

29. Gunnar MR, Frenn K, Wewerka SS, Van Ryzin MJ. Moderate versus severe early life stress: associations with stress reactivity and regulation in 10-12-year-old children. *Psychoneuroendocrinology.* 2009;34(1):62–75

30. Van Ryzin MJ, Chatham M, Kryzer E, Kertes DA, Gunnar MR. Identifying atypical cortisol patterns in young children: the benefits of group-based trajectory modeling. *Psychoneuroendocrinology.* 2009;34(1):50–61

31. Dozier M, Manni M, Gordon MK, et al. Foster children's diurnal production of cortisol: an exploratory study. *Child Maltreat.* 2006;11(2):189–197

32. Center on the Developing Child at Harvard University. Toxic stress. http://developingchild. harvard.edu/science/key-concepts/toxic-stress. Accessed February 27, 2018

33. Shonkoff JP, Garner AS; American Academy of Pediatrics Committee on Psychosocial Aspects of Child and Family Health; Committee on Early Childhood, Adoption, and Dependent Care; Section on Developmental and Behavioral Pediatrics. Technical report: the lifelong effects of early childhood adversity and toxic stress. *Pediatrics.* 2012;129(1):e232–e246

34. American Academy of Pediatrics Committee on Psychosocial Aspects of Child and Family Health; Committee on Early Childhood, Adoption, and Dependent Care; Section on Developmental and Behavioral Pediatrics. Policy statement: early childhood adversity, toxic stress, and the role of the pediatrician: translating developmental science into lifelong health. *Pediatrics.* 2012;129(1):e224–e231

Chapter 3

Epigenetics

· ·

We are the sum total of our experiences.

— *Thomas Gilovich*

· ·

Scientists and the lay public have long marveled and, at times, argued about the relative influences of genes and the environment on child development. Does one's genetic makeup, the inherited genome, ultimately determine one's destiny? Do various environmental influences affect the expression of these genes? In this age-old nature versus nurture debate, numerous examples point to an inextricable combination. For example, identical twins share the same set of genes, but diseases like diabetes mellitus and birth defects like cleft lip/palate often affect one twin and not the other. In one famous case, identical twins were switched at birth and raised as fraternal twins[1]; when reunited, the adult twins demonstrated dramatic similarities yet some ironic differences. These examples indicate that genes and the environment both matter,[2] but until recently, it was unclear how they interacted at the molecular level.

Recent advances from the burgeoning field of epigenetics make it clear that genes do not equal destiny, in part because the environment influences which sections of the DNA blueprint are actually used. *Epigenetics* literally means "above the genome" and refers to changes in gene expression that are *not* caused by changes in the DNA sequence itself. Through epigenetic changes, environmental factors (ie, experiences that happen to us) may turn genes off, turn genes on, or modulate them like a dimmer light switch. These epigenetic processes and their outcomes are now at the forefront of our understanding of how experiences become biologically embedded, and they are the focus of this chapter.

The Basics of Epigenetics

Background

In 1942, Conrad Waddington coined the term *epigenotype* to refer to the complex interactions that occur between the *genotype* (the DNA sequence in the genome) and the environment.[3] A *phenotype*, or a specific characteristic like a biochemical change, anatomic structure, or behavior, is the product of these complex interactions. As shown in Figure 3-1, we now understand there is more than a simple, causal, straight-line relationship between genotype and phenotype. The paradigm

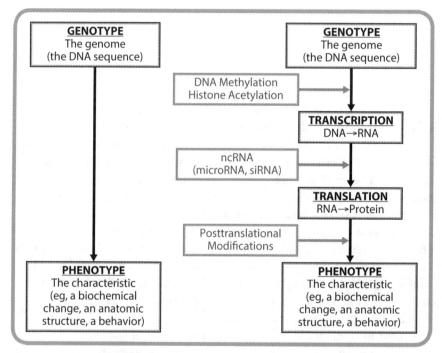

Figure 3-1. The complicated relationship between genotype and phenotype. *Genotype* refers to the specific DNA sequence within the genome. *Phenotype* refers to a characteristic attributed to the gene's protein product, be it a biochemical change, an anatomic structure, or even a behavior. The left side of the figure shows the classic model of genotype-to-phenotype determination. The right side shows the intervening steps between the gene and its expression as a phenotype: transcription, translation, and posttranslational modifications to the protein product of the gene. Additional factors regulating this progression from DNA to RNA to protein are shown in gray, and these are now known to be influenced by the environment. (Abbreviations: ncRNA, noncoding RNA, or RNA transcripts that do not code for protein products; microRNA, short sequences of ncRNA; siRNA, short interfering RNA.)

of genotype-to-phenotype is affected by environmental factors, random events, and interactive epigenetic factors, making the use of the genotype (the initial blueprint) to predict the phenotype (the final outcome) fraught with errors.[4] For example, every one of an individual's cells has the same DNA, yet some become liver cells, others become kidney cells, and still others become any of a multitude of other specialized cells. Rather than the genes *contained* in the cell, it is the genes *expressed* in that cell that determine its identity, and that panel of expressed genes is determined, in part, by the environmental factors that turn certain genes off or on. It is through this process that developmental lineages are defined and developmental potentials are restricted toward specific purposes. Although the process of cell differentiation or specialization is not entirely governed by epigenetic factors, those factors clearly play a pivotal role.

The rise of noncommunicable diseases, like hypertension, coronary artery disease (CAD), and non–insulin-dependent diabetes mellitus (NIDDM), is another case in which environmental and epigenetic factors are thought to play important roles. In 1990, British epidemiologist David J. P. Barker proposed that intrauterine growth retardation, low birth weight, and preterm birth are causally related to the development of hypertension, CAD, and NIDDM in adulthood (the so-called Barker hypothesis).[5] At the time, he was ridiculed because there were no known mechanisms to explain how events happening early in life could become biologically embedded and affect health outcomes decades later. Today, however, this phenomenon is well established, and the epigenetic mechanisms discussed in this chapter likely play a role. Barker's observation also underscores the point that the powerful dance between nature and nurture has the potential to swing in both directions. The complex interactions between the environment and the genotype can prove to be adaptive, better preparing the child for the future, but they can also be maladaptive and predispose the child to problems in physical and/or behavioral health later in childhood or adulthood.

Mechanisms

Three primary mechanisms are involved in modifying DNA expression without inducing DNA mutations (ie, without changing the DNA sequence): histone modification, DNA methylation, and noncoding RNA (ncRNA) (see Figure 3-1).

Histones are DNA-binding proteins that assist in the compaction of the long DNA molecule within the nucleus. The modification of histones by a variety of chemical reactions (eg, methylation, acetylation) can alter the protein's tertiary structure (or conformation), thereby turning genes on or off by altering the likelihood of transcription.

DNA methylation adds a $-CH_3$ group to cytosine bases within the DNA molecule and provides a mechanism for longer-lasting (but not necessarily permanent) changes in gene regulation. DNA methylation is predominantly associated with gene silencing (ie, turning genes off). Assays for DNA methylation are often used as a measure of epigenetic changes (ie, changes in the pattern presumably reflect changes in gene activation or deactivation).

Noncoding RNAs (or RNA molecules that do not code for protein products) also play an integral role in gene regulation, as microRNAs and short interfering RNAs bind to other transcripts and prevent their translation into protein. Interestingly, most of the DNA in the genome would be transcribed into ncRNA; the preservation of this noncoding DNA suggests that it plays an important role in overall genomic function.

The effects of turning a gene on or off will depend on the activity or role of the gene's product or protein. Certain gene products can be harmful when they are actively expressed (eg, oncogenes), whereas other gene products cause problems only when they are silenced (eg, tumor suppressors). The point here is that turning a gene on or off is not inherently good or bad; epigenetic changes simply alter the ability of a particular gene to be expressed, for better or for worse.

One noteworthy example of epigenetic gene regulation is the process known as *imprinting*, or the differential expression of genes based on the parent of origin. In genomic imprinting, the genes on all or part of a chromosome are modified differently depending on whether the chromosome came from the mother or father. As a consequence, the expression of genes will be different depending on which chromosome (maternal or paternal) is being used. The usual epigenetic modification seen with genomic imprinting is methylation, but histone modification and ncRNAs can both contribute. The biological utility of imprinting is still unclear, but its persistence suggests that it is likely to confer an evolutionary advantage.

Imprinted genes and imprinted gene regions are maintained throughout the life span of the somatic cell. This imprinting pattern is erased during the generation of primordial germ cells (the cells that lead to sperm in males and eggs in females), but it is reset after fertilization. Depending on whether the imprint is maternal or paternal, this erasure/restoration process occurs in different ways and to different degrees. The implications of these differing processes are still unknown.

The sum of these epigenetic mechanisms—histones, methylation, ncRNAs, imprinting, imprinting erasure, and imprinting restoration—is exquisite regulation of which genes are and are not expressed. While the terminology and concepts discussed herein might seem esoteric and confusing, their introduction in brief is critical to emphasize the main point that changes in gene expression without changes in the DNA sequence are the hallmark of epigenetics. The exact mechanisms underlying all the epigenetic sites of regulation throughout an individual's genome, known as that individual's *epigenome*, remain to be determined, but it is clear that the epigenome is alterable throughout one's lifetime. Epigenetic changes are evidence that genes are not destiny, that the early childhood ecology can be biologically embedded within the epigenome, and that subsequent events can also alter the way that the genetic blueprint is used.

Known Effects of Epigenetics

Historical Precedents

Numerous historical cases have shown how nutrition, or lack thereof, in the womb can affect gene expression. Infants exposed to in utero malnutrition during the Dutch famine at the end of World War II had an increased frequency of neural tube defects and schizophrenia.[6] Epigenetic changes (specifically, methylation patterns) were subsequently found to have differentially affected these offspring when compared with their control siblings, who were not exposed to famine in utero. What is even more intriguing is that in follow-up studies 60 years later, these epigenetic differences were found to persist between the exposed and unexposed siblings.

In another unfortunate social disaster, an increased risk of schizophrenia was found for children who were in utero during the Chinese famine in 1959 to 1961.[7] Epigenetic changes observed in similar situations in Gambia (different crop harvests based on rainfall)[8] and Sweden (different crop harvests depending on the weather during the growing season)[9] have also verified that altered food availability due to environmental conditions affects children and, potentially, their offspring for years to come. Interestingly, the changes in the Gambian experience appear to be related to maternal exposure, yet the changes in the Swedish experience appear to be related to paternal exposure.

Twin Studies

Epigenetic differences in monozygotic, or identical, twins have been found to be negligible at birth. However, up to one-third of monozygotic twins have documented differences in methylation or histone modification in adulthood.[10] Anecdotal stories of monozygotic twins[1,11] have noted similarities suggestive of shared innate abilities, yet different life experiences have led to differences in behavior and disease expression. In these circumstances, epigenetic changes are presumed to be at play.

Genetic Disorders

A variety of genetic disorders have been found or postulated to have epigenetic mechanisms (Box 3-1).[12] These disorders might also have a single gene etiology, demonstrating that various genetic and epigenetic factors can lead to a final common pathway or phenotype (eg, gene deletion, gene mutation, or reduced gene transcription due to DNA methylation could all lead to the inadequate expression of a particular gene product or protein).

Prader-Willi syndrome and Angelman syndrome are classic examples of genetic disorders that involve epigenetic mechanisms. Both of these disorders have some degree of intellectual disability, but the rest of their phenotypes are quite different. Although more standard, mutational etiologies are the most common causes of these disorders, imprinting plays a role as well. For example, inheriting 2 maternal copies of a certain region of chromosome 15q (effectively a paternal deletion) will lead to Prader-Willi syndrome, while 2 paternal copies of this imprinted region (effectively a maternal deletion) will lead to Angelman syndrome.[4,13] This mechanism

Box 3-1. Genetic Syndromes With Known or Putative Epigenetic Etiology

Angelman syndrome
Autism spectrum disorder
Beckwith-Wiedemann syndrome
CHARGE association
Fragile X syndrome
Maternal duplication 15q11-13
Metabolic syndrome
Prader-Willi syndrome
Rett syndrome
Silver-Russell syndrome
Turner syndrome

From Wright R, Saul RA. Epigenetics and primary care. *Pediatrics.* 2013;132(Suppl 3):S216–S223.

highlights the ability of epigenetic mechanisms to explain complex biological phenomena, like alterations in one gene locus leading to 2 very distinct genetic disorders.

Early Stress

Studies by Tyrka et al found that early life stress (ie, toxic stress) rendered demonstrable epigenetic changes.[14] The loss of a parent during childhood, maltreatment, and low parental care were associated with methylation changes to the promoter region of the glucocorticoid receptor (GR) gene *NR3C1*. Although these changes were noted in leucocytes, they are presumed to be generalizable to the central nervous system, where this receptor plays a major role in modulating the nervous system's response to stress (see Chapter 2). Methylation of the promoter region of this gene results in fewer GRs and is linked to alterations in the functioning of the hypothalamic-pituitary-adrenal axis and the body's flight or fight response. These findings suggest that early life stress can change a young child's pattern of DNA methylation, predisposing that child to altered stress responses and behavioral/developmental problems early in life. Maternal depression in the third trimester of pregnancy has produced similar findings.[15]

A related finding has been found in the postmortem analysis of the hippocampus in male suicide victims with a history of childhood abuse.[16] These specimens were compared with those from suicide victims who had not suffered childhood abuse and control subjects who had expired from unrelated causes. The suicide/abuse victims had increased methylation of the *NR3C1* promoter, and they had decreased levels of GR messenger RNA compared with the other groups. These findings were interpreted to suggest that childhood abuse might result in decreased expression of the GR gene and decreased activity of hippocampal GR in humans, possibly leading to a decrease in the child's ability to modulate the stress response.

Early prenatal influences also appear to have an effect. Cao-Lei and associates have used the Quebec ice storm of 1998 to record prenatal maternal self-assessment about coping mechanisms during a natural disaster (with possible concomitant maternal depression).[17] When measuring the methylation status across the genome in the subjects' offspring 13 years later, it appeared that pregnant women's cognitive appraisals of an independent stressor (ie, the ice storm) had effects on DNA methylation in their unborn children that were detectable during the children's adolescence. Therefore, cognitive appraisals could be an important factor in the assessment of children, as well as a potential measure for future interventions.

Early Nurturing

A study of a specific group of mothers found an astonishingly positive effect of maternal stroking of infants. Following up on experimental evidence demonstrating the positive effects of maternal licking in animals, Murgatroyd et al measured maternal stroking (by self-report) at 5 and 9 weeks after birth.[18] Significant maternal stroking was found to make a difference in the methylation of the GR gene in infants whose mothers had histories of low prenatal depression and subsequent elevated postnatal depression. If the mothers had increased maternal postnatal depression following low prenatal depression, the methylation in the promoter region was elevated, like the child abuse victims noted previously. Yet this effect was reversed by self-reported stroking, implying a reversible or protective effect of enhanced maternal nurturing. These findings (which will hopefully be replicated in future studies) offer direct evidence that parental nurturing can enhance positive epigenetic effects and diminish negative ones.

Implications for Health

Multiple factors have been identified to have epigenetic consequences (Box 3-2). These changes may be protective or harmful, depending on the time of exposure and their effects on gene expression and related biochemical processes. Figure 3-2 illustrates the susceptible periods for epigenetic changes

Box 3-2. Factors Leading to Epigenetic Changes

Diet during the slow-growth period
Hypoxia
Chemical exposures (eg, prenatal exposure to valproate)
Psychological trauma (post-traumatic stress disorder, depression)
Asthma (including allergic diseases)
Maternal diabetes
Endocrine-disrupting compounds (eg, bisphenol A)
Maternal smoking
Maternal habitus, maternal age, and placenta size

From Wright R, Saul RA. Epigenetics and primary care. *Pediatrics*. 2013;132(Suppl 3):S216–S223.

during the life cycle. Nutrition, uteroplacental factors, and maternal behavior are particularly critical.

The fact that such a wide variety of factors can lead to epigenetic changes through methylation, histone changes, or ncRNAs speaks to the need to consider many facets of the environment as we consider the factors to which our children are exposed prenatally and postnatally. The ecology of childhood is critical to a child's development and can have dramatic effects. Neither genes alone nor epigenetic changes alone define one's destiny.

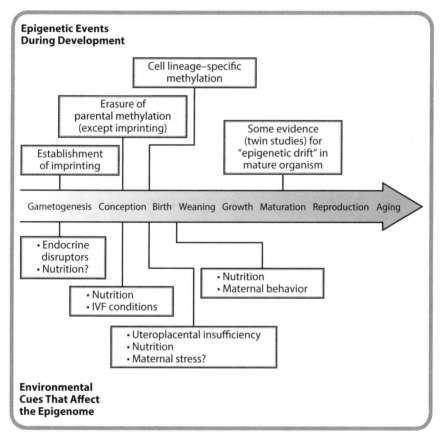

Figure 3-2. Timeline with susceptible periods for epigenetic changes. The events that occur naturally (establishment of imprinting, erasure of parental methylation except imprinting, cell-line–specific methylation, "epigenetic drift") are shown above the timeline. Environmental cues that can affect the epigenome are depicted below. (Abbreviation: IVF, in vitro fertilization.)

Adapted by permission from Springer Nature: Gluckman PD, Hanson MA, Buldijas T, et al. Epigenetic mechanisms that underpin metabolic and cardiovascular diseases. *Nat Rev Endocrinol.* 2009;5(7):401–408. Copyright 2009.

Adding Epigenetics to the Emerging Model

Figure 3-3 adds epigenetics to the emerging model of how the early childhood ecology affects developmental outcomes across the life span. Through epigenetic mechanisms, the early childhood ecology may become biologically embedded, leading to changes in the way the genetic blueprint is used. While the specific epigenetic mechanisms discussed in this chapter might seem esoteric or irrelevant to parents, teachers, or clinical practice, a basic understanding of epigenetics is needed to appreciate how childhood experiences become biologically embedded and lead to changes in the functioning of the genome. Epigenetic mechanisms begin to explain what is going on inside the proverbial black box: childhood experiences, both adverse (eg, maternal depression, child

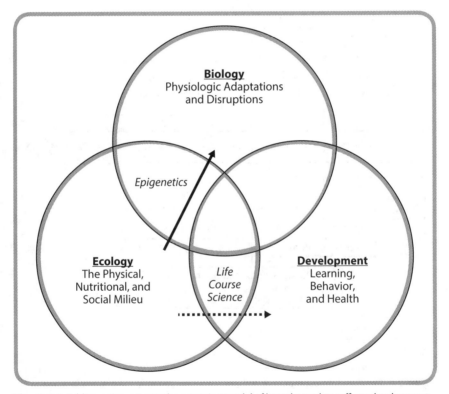

Figure 3-3. Adding epigenetics to the emerging model of how the ecology affects development. Life course science has repeatedly demonstrated strong associations (dotted arrow) between the early childhood ecology and developmental outcomes in learning, behavior, and health. Through epigenetic mechanisms, the early childhood ecology is biologically embedded (solid arrow), leading to changes in the way the genetic blueprint is used.

maltreatment) and affiliative (maternal-infant stroking), lead to changes in the genome. To understand how these changes, in turn, affect learning, behavior, and health decades later, a familiarity with the basic mechanisms and principles of brain development are required. These mechanisms and principles are discussed in the next chapter.

References

1. Dominus S. The mixed-up brothers of Bogota. *New York Times Magazine*. July 9, 2015. https://www.nytimes.com/2015/07/12/magazine/the-mixed-up-brothers-of-bogota.html. Accessed February 27, 2018

2. Gluckman PD, Hanson MA, Cooper C, Thornburg KL. Effect of in utero and early-life conditions on adult health and disease. *N Engl J Med*. 2008;359(1):61–73

3. Waddington CH. The epigenotype. 1942. *Int J Epidemiol*. 2012;41(1):10–13

4. Parisi MA. Genetics over the life cycle. In: Saul RA, ed. *Medical Genetics in Pediatric Practice*. Elk Grove Village, IL: American Academy of Pediatrics; 2013:21–49

5. Barker DJ. The fetal and infant origins of adult disease. *BMJ*. 1990;301(6761):1111

6. Heijmans BT, Tobi EW, Stein AD, et al. Persistent epigenetic differences associated with prenatal exposure to famine in humans. *Proc Natl Acad Sci U S A*. 2008;105(44):17046–17049

7. St Clair D, Xu M, Wang P, et al. Rates of adult schizophrenia following prenatal exposure to the Chinese famine of 1959-1961. *JAMA*. 2005;294(5):557–562

8. Waterland RA, Kellermayer R, Laritsky E, et al. Season of conception in rural Gambia affects DNA methylation at putative human metastable epialleles. *PLoS Genet*. 2010;6(12):e1001252

9. Kaati G, Bygren LO, Pembrey M, Sjöström M. Transgenerational response to nutrition, early life circumstances and longevity. *Eur J Hum Genet*. 2007;15(7):784–790

10. Fraga MF, Ballestar E, Paz MF, et al. Epigenetic differences arise during the lifetime of monozygotic twins. *Proc Natl Acad Sci U S A*. 2005;102(30):10604–10609

11. Mukherjee S. Same but different. *The New Yorker*. May 2, 2016. https://www.newyorker.com/magazine/2016/05/02/breakthroughs-in-epigenetics. Accessed February 27, 2018

12. Wright R, Saul RA. Epigenetics and primary care. *Pediatrics*. 2013;132(Suppl 3):S216–S223

13. Lyons MJ. Specific genetic conditions. In: Saul RA, ed. *Medical Genetics in Pediatric Practice*. Elk Grove Village, IL: American Acadey of Pediatrics; 2013:175–234

14. Tyrka AR, Price LH, Marsit C, Walters OC, Carpenter LL. Childhood adversity and epigenetic modulation of the leukocyte glucocorticoid receptor: preliminary findings in healthy adults. *PLoS One*. 2012;7(1):e30148

15. Oberlander TF, Weinberg J, Papsdorf M, Grunau R, Misri S, Devlin AM. Prenatal exposure to maternal depression, neonatal methylation of human glucocorticoid receptor gene (NR3C1) and infant cortisol stress responses. *Epigenetics*. 2008;3(2):97–106

16. McGowan PO, Sasaki A, D'Alessio AC, et al. Epigenetic regulation of the glucocorticoid receptor in human brain associates with childhood abuse. *Nat Neurosci*. 2009;12(3):342–348

17. Cao-Lei L, Dancause KN, Elgbeili G, et al. DNA methylation mediates the impact of exposure to prenatal maternal stress on BMI and central adiposity in children at age 13½ years: Project Ice Storm. *Epigenetics*. 2015;10(8):749–761

18. Murgatroyd C, Quinn JP, Sharp HM, Pickles A, Hill J. Effects of prenatal and postnatal depression, and maternal stroking, at the glucocorticoid receptor gene. *Transl Psychiatry*. 2015;5:e560

Chapter 4

Developmental Neuroscience

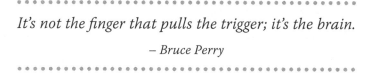

It's not the finger that pulls the trigger; it's the brain.

– *Bruce Perry*

Epigenetics allows us to peer inside the black box and better understand how experiences in childhood, both affiliative and adverse, are able to influence outcomes in learning, behavior, and health decades later. Through epigenetic mechanisms, early experiences are biologically embedded and influence which parts of the genetic blueprint are actually read and utilized. Another way that experiences are biologically embedded lies in their ability to alter the structure and function of the developing brain. To understand how early childhood adversity and toxic stress alter brain structure and function in a potentially permanent manner, one must first appreciate the cellular mechanisms and basic principles of typical brain development. This chapter will briefly describe 3 cellular mechanisms and 5 overarching principles of brain development before considering how toxic stress and early adversity leave their mark on brain structure and function.

Three Basic Mechanisms Underlying Brain Development

To say that the development of the human brain is complicated is an understatement. Consider just the numbers. At conception, the soon-to-be fetus is a single, solitary cell. But the adult brain consists of several billion neurons[1] with trillions of connections or synapses.[2] In this context, it is amazing that any 2 humans are even remotely alike. And these numbers do not include the other cells of the brain, like astrocytes, oligodendrocytes, and microglia, whose functions are also critically important for brain development and function. For our purposes here, however, we will focus primarily on neuronal development and 3 basic mechanisms: generating the number of neurons, determining their connections, and increasing their speed of communication (Figure 4-1).

Number of Neurons

The number of neurons in the brain is the net result of neuronal production (neurogenesis) and neuronal loss (apoptosis or programmed cell death). Neurogenesis occurs primarily before birth. Although there are a few notable exceptions,[3] the vast majority of neurons in an adult brain, about 80 billion,[1] were present at birth. But not all the neurons that were generated in utero survive until birth; many are eliminated through programmed cell death.[4–6] At first blush, this might seem like a wasteful way to build a brain. Consider, though, the way artists fashion a sculpture or carving: they begin with an excess of material to ensure completeness, and then slowly and carefully eliminate what is no longer needed. Although the vast majority of neurogenesis occurs in utero, there is limited, ongoing neurogenesis in select areas of the brain, like the hippocampus.[3] The hippocampus is critically important for

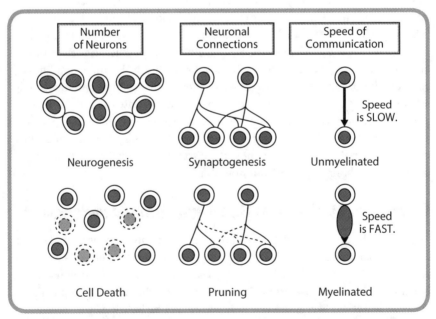

Figure 4-1. Neuronal development is a function of the number of neurons, their connections, and their speed of communication. The number of neurons is the result of *neurogenesis,* which occurs primarily in utero, and programmed *cell death.* Similarly, the number of neuronal connections is the product of *synaptogenesis* and *pruning.* Finally, the speed of communication is dependent on *myelination* because the fatty sheath of myelin provided by oligodendrocytes dramatically increases the speed of signal transduction along the axon.

learning and memory, and the addition of new neurons to this structure is thought to contribute to its *plasticity*—its ability to change with experience.[7]

Neuronal Connections

Overproduction to ensure completeness, followed by pruning to eliminate what is not needed, is a motif also seen in the generation of the connections, or *synapses*, between the neurons. By 18 months of age, the number of synapses in the brain is thought to be in the hundreds of trillions.[2] Many of these synapses occur in the so-called gray matter that covers the surfaces of the brain. But by 3 years of age, many of these synapses have been pruned. This pruning continues throughout childhood and thins the gray matter, leaving only the most frequently used connections in place. Recent studies using serial, noninvasive imaging techniques, like magnetic resonance imaging, have demonstrated that this process of synaptogenesis followed by pruning occurs again in early adolescence.[8] Researchers have speculated that this may be one last attempt to get the wiring finely tuned for adult functioning.

Neuronal Myelination

Once the neurons are generated and have connected via synapses, the signal-sending axons of the neurons are wrapped in a fatty sheath called *myelin*. This process, called *myelination*, dramatically speeds up the electrical impulse of the neuron's axons, so individual neurons can communicate with each other more quickly.[9] As a result, a network of myelinated neurons is able to process information and initiate responses more swiftly. Because myelin appears white on cross sections of the brain, myelination results in more white matter. Myelination is an important measure of maturity, and some structures in the brain are not completely myelinated or structurally mature until 24 years of age.[8]

Five Overarching Principles of Brain Development

The 1990s were declared the "Decade of the Brain" by the National Institutes of Health.[10] As part of this initiative, significant investments were made into advancing our understanding of how the brain is assembled. Although a comprehensive discussion of the molecular mechanisms underlying brain development is beyond the scope of this discussion, it is worth noting 5 overarching principles. In short, brain development is
1. Experience dependent
2. Cumulative
3. Integrated
4. Dynamic
5. Asynchronous

Understanding these 5 principles, along with the 3 basic mechanisms of brain development described previously, will allow for a more sophisticated discussion of how adversity becomes biologically embedded (Table 4-1).

Principle #1: Experience Dependent

Above all else, brain development is experience dependent. Although the genetic blueprint is known to play an important role in directing the basic architecture of the brain, experiences and the neuronal activity they generate are absolutely necessary for proper brain development and function. A classic example comes from the Nobel Prize–winning work of Hubel and Wiesel.[11–17] They demonstrated that the normal architecture of the primary visual cortex consists of ocular dominance columns, where groups of neurons respond only to the visual stimulation from one eye. However, this normal architecture and responsiveness is irreversibly altered simply by preventing one eye from transmitting visual experiences to the brain. The neuronal activity generated in the cortex by visual experience is absolutely necessary for the normal development of the ocular dominance columns. This important work led to a deeper understanding of amblyopia, a condition where the brain eventually stops responding to the electrical signals coming from a weaker eye.

The experience dependence of brain development is not surprising given that experiences and the neuronal activity generated by experiences influence all 3 of the cellular mechanisms described earlier.[18–28] In particular, experience and neuronal activity play an important role in generating new synapses (synaptogenesis) and in determining which synapses are maintained (not pruned).[22,29] This has led to the aphorisms that "neurons that fire together, wire together" and "if you don't use it [the synapse], you lose it."

Because brain development is experience dependent, it is useful to think about different parts of the brain as muscles: The parts that are used frequently are strengthened over time. The question then becomes which parts of the brain are being strengthened by early experiences. Are affiliative childhood experiences strengthening the brain structures necessary for behaviors like social interactions, language skills, emotional regulation, and sustained attention? Or are adverse experiences instead strengthening the brain structures that drive impulsive or aggressive behaviors, like flight or fight? Early social experiences play a pivotal role in determining which brain structures, behaviors, and skills are strengthened over time.[30–32]

Principle #2: Cumulative

Much like a building, the brain is built from the bottom up. Simple synapses between neurons lead to basic circuits, which are integrated into

Table 4-1. Brief Descriptions of 5 Principles of Brain Development and Their Clinical Significance

General Principles	Description	Significance
Experience dependent	Experiences (and the neuronal activity they generate) sculpt brain development by changing the number of neurons, number of neuronal connections, and speed of neuronal communication.	The brain is like a muscle. Which neuronal pathways and brain structures are being reinforced and strengthened by early experiences?
Cumulative	Brain development is cumulative because synapses are the building blocks for neuronal pathways, which, in turn, are the building blocks for complex brain functions, like cognition and behavior.	Like a building, the brain is built from the bottom up. Are early experiences forging a strong or weak foundation for future growth?
Integrated	To understand the brain, we often look at discrete domains like cognitive skills versus social or language skills. But the brain is more like an intricate spiderweb, and deficits in one domain may lead to deficits in another.	Brain development is like playing solitaire: If you are missing one of the aces (eg, social-emotional skills), progress is more difficult.
Dynamic	Synaptic and cellular plasticity allow the brain to reorganize itself in response to experiences. But cellular plasticity declines with age, making it harder to teach an old dog new tricks.	Declining brain plasticity underscores the importance of getting early experiences and brain connectivity right the first time.
Asynchronous	Different structures in the brain (and the functions that those structures serve) mature at different rates. For example, the prefrontal cortex is not structurally mature until 24 years of age, whereas the amygdala is structurally mature much earlier.	Because the "on switch" for the body's stress response matures sooner than the "off switch," early life adversity may promote toxic stress responses.

In the Cumulative row illustration: Cognition and Behavior, Neuronal Pathways, Synapses

In the Dynamic row illustration: Difficulty of change increases. Cellular plasticity declines.

In the Asynchronous row illustration: Matures later / OFF; ON / Matures sooner more complex pathways, which culminate in behavior and thought. Consequently, the earliest, most foundational connections in the brain are critical. Early skills lead to more complex skills, but early deficits often lead to more deficits.[33]

A classic example of this principle comes from the work of Hart and Risley, who compared the word exposures and vocabularies of children from wealthy and impoverished families.[34,35] During the first 4 years after birth (ending at the child's fourth birthday), children in the wealthy families were exposed to almost 45 million words, whereas the children in impoverished families were exposed to only 13 million words. This so-called 30-million–word gap was associated with dramatic differences in the children's vocabulary. Disparities in vocabulary between children in the 2 groups appeared as early as 18 months of age, and these disparities only widened over time. The work of Hart and Risley demonstrates that early experiences are foundational and cumulative, setting the stage for future success or failure.

Principle #3: Integrated

It has been said that the human brain is "the most complicated 3-pound mass of matter in the universe."[8] In our attempts to understand this complexity, we tend to parse out one skill from another. For example, we may consider cognitive skills to be distinct from language skills, social skills, emotional skills, or the regulation of attention. While it is true that discrete areas of the brain appear to be more necessary for certain skills than others, the brain is more like a complex spiderweb, with most areas being inextricably connected to many others.[33] Perhaps this is not surprising, given that most of human behavior requires the use of multiple skill sets at the same time. For example, academic achievement tests may be designed to measure learned material, but they also require language and reading skills to understand the directions, social skills to have the motivation and confidence to try, emotional skills to deal with the frustration of not knowing all the answers, and attentional skills to remain focused on a task that might not be terribly exciting. In this sense, brain development is like playing a game of solitaire: If you do not have all the aces, you will only get so far. Optimal early brain and child development demands the integration and use of a full complement of cognitive, language, social, emotional, and attentional skills.

In addition to highlighting the importance of whole child development and education, the brain's almost inextricable integration makes the relationship between structure and function fraught with peril. For example, throughout this book, we will attribute certain brain functions to specific brain structures: the amygdala as an *on* switch for the body's stress response; the amygdala as an inhibitor of the prefrontal cortex and hippocampus; the prefrontal cortex and hippocampus as *off* switches for the body's stress response; and the prefrontal cortex and hippocampus as critical structures for learning and adaptive behaviors. While these general attributions are certainly true, the amygdala, prefrontal cortex, and hippocampus are known to play important roles in many other pathways and behaviors as well. In addition, there are discrete clusters of neurons within each of these larger structures that behave in unusual ways (eg, amygdala neurons that *activate* the prefrontal cortex and hippocampus rather than inhibiting them). For a more in-depth and nuanced look at these important brain structures and their microanatomy, numerous connections, and attributed functions, see Robert Sapolsky's book *Behave: The Biology of Humans at Our Best and Worst.*[36]

Principle #4: Dynamic

Experiences drive not only the initial wiring of the brain but also the brain's ongoing ability to rewire itself in a dynamic manner based on the demands of the environment. As previously mentioned, this ability is called *plasticity,*[9] and there are 2 distinct types: synaptic and cellular. *Synaptic plasticity* refers to the ability of experience to change the *strength* of individual synapses between neurons. Synaptic plasticity is like turning up the volume of a speaker: a synapse can serve as a whisper between 2 cells, or it can act like one neuron is shouting at the other. Synaptic plasticity is thought to be lifelong, allowing even old dogs to learn new tricks.

Cellular plasticity refers to the ability of experience to change the *number* of synapses between 2 neurons. Cellular plasticity is like going from one person shouting to a stadium full of people shouting and is, therefore, a much more powerful form of plasticity. Cellular plasticity is greatest in early childhood. Unfortunately, much of the brain's cellular plasticity is waning by the time children enter school.[31] This time course underscores the importance of setting a strong foundational architecture for the brain early in life, before cellular plasticity begins to wane.[37] The persistence of synaptic plasticity means that ongoing, dynamic change is possible, but change is much harder as time goes on.

Principle #5: Asynchronous

Although the general progression from neurogenesis to synaptogenesis to myelination occurs throughout the brain, not all structures mature at the same rate.[31] Overall, brain maturation progresses from the back of the brain toward the front, and the maturation of brain regions parallels the developmental progression of the functions and behaviors that those regions are known to support.[8] For example, the structures important for vital processes (eg, the regulation of breathing, heart rate, and blood pressure), like those in the brain stem, are structurally mature at birth. Next, the visual cortex and parietal cortex mature, allowing for the visual tracking of objects, social smiles, and the integration of sensory and motor functions. Then, the structures of the limbic system mature, providing for the emotionality and tantrums frequently seen in toddlers. Fortunately, the temporal lobes mature shortly thereafter, allowing for the development of verbal language skills and (hopefully) the lessening of frustrations. The last area to mature is the prefrontal cortex, which is important for executive functioning and acts much like an air traffic controller for the brain.[38] The prefrontal cortex has been called the "seat of humanity"[39] because it allows for the abstract thought, planning, emotion regulation, and control of attention necessary for humans to imagine, create, and collaborate.

The differential maturation of brain structures (and the functions and behaviors they support) has important ramifications. Recall that the amygdala, the *on* switch for the flight or fight response, is part of the limbic system and matures relatively early when compared with the prefrontal cortex, which serves as an important *off* switch for the body's stress response. In fact, the prefrontal cortex is not completely myelinated and structurally mature until 24 years of age.[8] Throughout childhood and adolescence, the off switch for the stress response (prefrontal cortex) is still struggling to find its voice, while the on switch for the stress response (amygdala) starts shouting early in child development.[40]

From a survival standpoint, the differential maturation of the on switch and the off switch for the body's stress response makes sense. When young, it may be safer to "shoot first and ask questions later," or there may not *be* a later. Once the child is older and wiser and more competent at assessing risks, impulsive flight or fight reactions may no longer be the most prudent course of action.

Effect of Early Adversity on Brain Development

Having reviewed the 3 cellular mechanisms and 5 overarching principles of brain development, it should now be clear how early childhood adversity and toxic stress become biologically embedded. Toxic stress alters all 3 cellular mechanisms of brain development: the numbers, connections, and speed of communication. For example, significant adversity and chronic exposure to cortisol and other glucocorticoids prevents neurogenesis and promotes cell death in the hippocampus.[41–46] Glucocorticoids and stress alter synaptogenesis and the remodeling of the prefrontal cortex.[47–51] Finally, glucocorticoids alter myelination and the maturation of white matter structures.[52–54]

Because brain development is experience dependent, early adversities have the potential to alter the foundational architecture and ongoing remodeling of the brain. Because brain development is cumulative, disruptions and deficits caused by early adversities may set the stage for additional disruptions and deficits down the line. Because brain development is integrated, strong cognitive skills may be insufficient to overcome the deficits in social-emotional skills that are often associated with early adversity. Because brain development is dynamic, the opportunities to repair, remediate, and fix maladaptive alterations caused by early adversity decline with age.[31,37]

Finally, because brain development is asynchronous, early adversity can lead to a vicious cycle of toxic stress. Because the off switch is still finding its voice, early adversity can lead to a longer-term or chronic stress response.[55] Because of the plasticity of the young brain, the chronic stress response can lead to changes in brain architecture.[55] For example, orphans who have been institutionalized literally have a larger amygdala than other children their age.[56] But the adversity does not necessarily need to be catastrophic to have this effect; children born to mothers with depression also have changes in the size of the amygdala.[57] Because the amygdala inhibits the prefrontal cortex, children who have experienced early adversity or chronic stress are less able to activate their prefrontal cortex or to downregulate their stress response later in life.[58] Simply stated, toxic stress begets more toxic stress.

Adding Neuroscience to the Emerging Model

Figure 4-2 adds neuroscience to the emerging model of how the early childhood ecology affects developmental outcomes across the life span. Through epigenetic mechanisms, the early childhood ecology is biologically embedded, leading to changes in the way the genetic blueprint is used. The 3 basic mechanisms and 5 general principles of brain development discussed in this chapter allow us to better understand how early childhood ecology alters brain structure and function and, in turn, outcomes in behavior, learning, and health decades later. But it is important to note that the mediators of toxic stress responses, like cortisol, also alter the development and function of organs other than the brain. For example, cortisol is known to alter endocrine and immune function, leading to chronic changes that may underlie adult-manifest, noncommunicable diseases, like obesity, hypertension, cancer, and autoimmune disorders.[59]

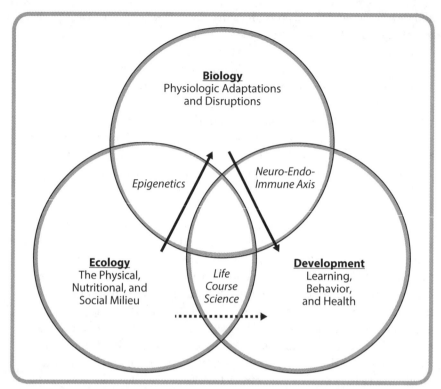

Figure 4-2. Adding developmental neuroscience to the emerging model of how the ecology affects development. Life course science has repeatedly demonstrated strong associations (dotted arrow) between the early childhood ecology and developmental outcomes in learning, behavior, and health. Through epigenetic mechanisms (solid arrow), the early childhood ecology is biologically embedded, leading to changes in the way the genetic blueprint is used. Developmental neuroscience helps us to understand how those biological changes (adaptive and disruptive) lead to alterations in brain structure/function and, ultimately, to differential outcomes in behavior, learning, and health (solid arrow). The neuro-endo-immune axis refers to the fact that the mediators of toxic stress responses (eg, cortisol) influence not only brain development but the functioning of the endocrine and immune systems, leading to chronic changes that may underlie conditions like obesity, hypertension, cancer, and autoimmune disorders.[59]

Effect of Safe, Stable, and Nurturing Relationships

From a neuroscience perspective, then, what is the antidote to early childhood adversity and toxic stress? It is safe, stable, and nurturing relationships (Figure 4-3). In the absence of safe, stable, and nurturing relationships, when the brain is in *survival mode*, toxic stress responses promote the function of the amygdala and inhibit the functioning of the prefrontal cortex and hippocampus, leading to more impulsive and aggressive behaviors and, ultimately, additional toxic stress. But in the presence of safe, stable, and nurturing relationships, when

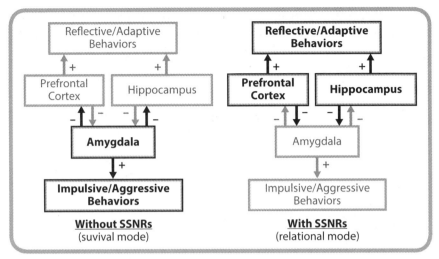

Figure 4-3. Safe, stable, and nurturing relationships (SSNRs) are the antidote to early childhood adversity and toxic stress responses. Without SSNRs (when in survival mode), early adversity leads to a strong amygdala, which inhibits the prefrontal cortex and hippocampus (black arrows). That inhibition, in turn, limits their ability to inhibit the amygdala and decreases the adoption of reflective/adaptive behaviors (gray arrows). But with SSNRs (when in relational mode), briefer and more moderate stress responses allow the prefrontal cortex and hippocampus to develop and strengthen over time. A strong prefrontal cortex and hippocampus promote reflective, adaptive behaviors and inhibit the amygdala (black arrows). This inhibition of the amygdala, in turn, limits its ability to inhibit the prefrontal cortex and hippocampus and decreases the adoption of impulsive or aggressive behaviors (gray arrows). In sum, SSNRs help to determine which brain structures tend to have the upper hand, the amygdala or the prefrontal cortex and hippocampus.

the brain is in *relational mode,* the brevity of the physiologic stress response to adversity turns off the amygdala, promotes the functioning of the prefrontal cortex and hippocampus, and leads to more reflective and adaptive behaviors. These adaptive behaviors, in turn, engender additional social supports and lead to less stress in the future. Early experiences help to shape this dynamic, ongoing balance between the amygdala and survival mode, on one hand, and the prefrontal cortex, hippocampus, and relational mode, on the other. Unabated adversity strengthens the amygdala and promotes impulsive, aggressive behaviors, like flight or fight, whereas safe, stable, and nurturing relationships strengthen the prefrontal cortex and hippocampus, allowing for more reflective, adaptive behaviors, like affiliate (see Figure 4-3).

The biology of toxic stress tells us that relational health, or the ability to form and maintain safe, stable, and nurturing relationships, is the antidote to significant childhood adversity. But to implement and disseminate this antidote, significant, even transformational changes are needed, not only in health care but in the education and social service systems. To promote this transformational change, a new model of health and wellness is needed. The next chapter discusses the evolution of models of health and the advantages of an ecobiodevelopmental model of disease and wellness.

References

1. Azevedo FA, Carvalho LR, Grinberg LT, et al. Equal numbers of neuronal and nonneuronal cells make the human brain an isometrically scaled-up primate brain. *J Comp Neurol.* 2009;513(5):532–541

2. Tang Y, Nyengaard JR, De Groot DM, Gundersen HJ. Total regional and global number of synapses in the human brain neocortex. *Synapse.* 2001;41(3):258–273

3. Bergmann O, Spalding KL, Frisén J. Adult neurogenesis in humans. *Cold Spring Harb Perspect Biol.* 2015;7(7):a018994

4. Hutchins JB, Barger SW. Why neurons die: cell death in the nervous system. *Anat Rec.* 1998;253(3):79–90

5. Monk CS, Webb SJ, Nelson CA. Prenatal neurobiological development: molecular mechanisms and anatomical change. *Dev Neuropsychol.* 2001;19(2):211–236

6. Dekkers MP, Nikoletopoulou V, Barde YA. Cell biology in neuroscience: death of developing neurons: new insights and implications for connectivity. *J Cell Biol.* 2013;203(3):385–393

7. Toni N, Schinder AF. Maturation and functional integration of new granule cells into the adult hippocampus. *Cold Spring Harb Perspect Biol.* 2015;8(1):a018903

8. Shaw P, Kabani NJ, Lerch JP, et al. Neurodevelopmental trajectories of the human cerebral cortex. *J Neurosci.* 2008;28(14):3586–3594

9. Kandel ER, Schwartz JH, Jessell TM, Siegelbaum SA, Hudspeth AJ, eds. *Principles of Neural Science.* 5th ed. New York, NY: McGraw-Hill Medical; 2013

10. Goldstein M. The Decade of the Brain: an era of promise for neurosurgery and a call to action. *J Neurosurg.* 1990;73(1):1–2

11. Hubel DH, Wiesel TN. The period of susceptibility to the physiological effects of unilateral eye closure in kittens. *J Physiol.* 1970;206(2):419–436

12. Wiesel TN, Hubel DH. Extent of recovery from the effects of visual deprivation in kittens. *J Neurophysiol.* 1965;28(6):1060–1072

13. Hubel DH, Wiesel TN. Binocular interaction in striate cortex of kittens reared with artificial squint. *J Neurophysiol.* 1965;28(6):1041–1059

14. Hubel DH, Wiesel TN. Effects of monocular deprivation in kittens. *Naunyn Schmiedebergs Arch Exp Pathol Pharmakol.* 1964;248:492–497

15. Wiesel TN, Hubel DH. Effects of visual deprivation on morphology and physiology of cells in the cats lateral geniculate body. *J Neurophysiol.* 1963;26:978–993

16. Wiesel TN, Hubel DH. Single-cell responses in striate cortex of kittens deprived of vision in one eye. *J Neurophysiol.* 1963;26:1003–1017

17. Hubel DH, Wiesel TN. Shape and arrangement of columns in cat's striate cortex. *J Physiol.* 1963;165:559–568

18. Kempermann G. Activity dependency and aging in the regulation of adult neurogenesis. *Cold Spring Harb Perspect Biol.* 2015;7(11):a018929

19. Klempin F, Beis D, Mosienko V, Kempermann G, Bader M, Alenina N. Serotonin is required for exercise-induced adult hippocampal neurogenesis. *J Neurosci.* 2013;33(19):8270–8275

20. Ma DK, Jang MH, Guo JU, et al. Neuronal activity-induced Gadd45b promotes epigenetic DNA demethylation and adult neurogenesis. *Science.* 2009;323(5917):1074–1077

21. Cesa R, Scelfo B, Strata P. Activity-dependent presynaptic and postsynaptic structural plasticity in the mature cerebellum. *J Neurosci.* 2007;27(17):4603–4611

22. Hu B, Nikolakopoulou AM, Cohen-Cory S. BDNF stabilizes synapses and maintains the structural complexity of optic axons in vivo. *Development.* 2005;132(19):4285–4298

23. Tian X, Kai L, Hockberger PE, Wokosin DL, Surmeier DJ. MEF-2 regulates activity-dependent spine loss in striatopallidal medium spiny neurons. *Mol Cell Neurosci.* 2010;44(1):94–108

24. Lee H, Brott BK, Kirkby LA, et al. Synapse elimination and learning rules co-regulated by MHC class I H2-Db. *Nature.* 2014;509(7499):195–200

25. Nikonenko I, Nikonenko A, Mendez P, Michurina TV, Enikolopov G, Muller D. Nitric oxide mediates local activity-dependent excitatory synapse development. *Proc Natl Acad Sci U S A.* 2013;110(44):E4142–E4151

26. Fields RD. A new mechanism of nervous system plasticity: activity-dependent myelination. *Nat Rev Neurosci.* 2015;16(12):756–767

27. Hines JH, Ravanelli AM, Schwindt R, Scott EK, Appel B. Neuronal activity biases axon selection for myelination in vivo. *Nat Neurosci.* 2015;18(5):683–689

28. Jensen SK, Yong VW. Activity-dependent and experience-driven myelination provide new directions for the management of multiple sclerosis. *Trends Neurosci.* 2016;39(6):356–365

29. Orefice LL, Shih CC, Xu H, Waterhouse EG, Xu B. Control of spine maturation and pruning through proBDNF synthesized and released in dendrites. *Mol Cell Neurosci.* 2016;71:66–79

30. Center on the Developing Child at Harvard University. *Supportive Relationships and Active Skill-Building Strengthen the Foundations of Resilience: Working Paper No. 13.* 2015. https://developingchild.harvard.edu/resources/supportive-relationships-and-active-skill-building-strengthen-the-foundations-of-resilience. Accessed February 28, 2018

31. National Scientific Council on the Developing Child. *The Timing and Quality of Early Experiences Combine to Shape Brain Architecture: Working Paper No. 5.* 2007. https://developingchild.harvard.edu/resources/the-timing-and-quality-of-early-experiences-combine-to-shape-brain-architecture. Accessed February 28, 2018

32. National Scientific Council on the Developing Child. *Young Children Develop in an Environment of Relationships: Working Paper No. 1.* 2004. https://developingchild.harvard.edu/resources/wp1. Accessed February 28, 2018

33. Center on the Developing Child at Harvard University. Brain architecture. 2010. https://developingchild.harvard.edu/science/key-concepts/brain-architecture. Accessed February 28, 2018

34. Hart B, Risley TR. *The Social World of Children Learning to Talk.* Baltimore, MD: Paul H. Brookes Publishing Co; 1999

35. Hart B, Risley TR. *Meaningful Differences in the Everyday Experience of Young American Children.* Baltimore, MD: Paul H. Brookes Publishing Co; 1995

36. Sapolsky RM. *Behave: The Biology of Humans at Our Best and Worst.* New York, NY: Penguin Press; 2017

37. Fox SE, Levitt P, Nelson CA 3rd. How the timing and quality of early experiences influence the development of brain architecture. *Child Dev.* 2010;81(1):28–40

38. Center on the Developing Child at Harvard University. *Building the Brain's "Air Traffic Control" System: How Early Experiences Shape the Development of Executive Function: Working Paper No. 11.* 2011. https://developingchild.harvard.edu/resources/building-the-brains-air-traffic-control-system-how-early-experiences-shape-the-development-of-executive-function. Accessed February 28, 2018

39. Sagan C. *Cosmos.* New York, NY: Random House; 1980

40. Gabard-Durnam LJ, Flannery J, Goff B, et al. The development of human amygdala functional connectivity at rest from 4 to 23 years: a cross-sectional study. *Neuroimage.* 2014;95:193–207

41. Lee AL, Ogle WO, Sapolsky RM. Stress and depression: possible links to neuron death in the hippocampus. *Bipolar Disord.* 2002;4(2):117–128

42. McEwen BS. Plasticity of the hippocampus: adaptation to chronic stress and allostatic load. *Ann N Y Acad Sci.* 2001;933:265–277

43. Conrad CD. Chronic stress-induced hippocampal vulnerability: the glucocorticoid vulnerability hypothesis. *Rev Neurosci.* 2008;19(6):395–411

44. Fitzsimons CP, Herbert J, Schouten M, Meijer OC, Lucassen PJ, Lightman S. Circadian and ultradian glucocorticoid rhythmicity: implications for the effects of glucocorticoids on neural stem cells and adult hippocampal neurogenesis. *Front Neuroendocrinol.* 2016;41:44–58

45. Lucassen PJ, Oomen CA, Naninck EF, et al. Regulation of adult neurogenesis and plasticity by (early) stress, glucocorticoids, and inflammation. *Cold Spring Harb Perspect Biol.* 2015;7(9):a021303

46. Schoenfeld TJ, Gould E. Stress, stress hormones, and adult neurogenesis. *Exp Neurol.* 2012;233(1):12–21

47. Fuchs E, Flugge G, Czeh B. Remodeling of neuronal networks by stress. *Front Biosci.* 2006;11:2746–2758

48. McEwen BS. The ever-changing brain: cellular and molecular mechanisms for the effects of stressful experiences. *Dev Neurobiol.* 2012;72(6):878–890

49. Musazzi L, Treccani G, Popoli M. Functional and structural remodeling of glutamate synapses in prefrontal and frontal cortex induced by behavioral stress. *Front Psychiatry.* 2015;6:60

50. Popoli M, Yan Z, McEwen BS, Sanacora G. The stressed synapse: the impact of stress and glucocorticoids on glutamate transmission. *Nat Rev Neurosci.* 2011;13(1):22–37

51. Butts KA, Weinberg J, Young AH, Phillips AG. Glucocorticoid receptors in the prefrontal cortex regulate stress-evoked dopamine efflux and aspects of executive function. *Proc Natl Acad Sci U S A.* 2011;108(45):18459–18464

52. Tomlinson L, Leiton CV, Colognato H. Behavioral experiences as drivers of oligodendrocyte lineage dynamics and myelin plasticity. *Neuropharmacology.* 2016;110(Pt B):548–562

53. Lyons DM, Parker KJ, Katz M, Schatzberg AF. Developmental cascades linking stress inoculation, arousal regulation, and resilience. *Front Behav Neurosci.* 2009;3:32

54. Chetty S, Friedman AR, Taravosh-Lahn K, et al. Stress and glucocorticoids promote oligodendrogenesis in the adult hippocampus. *Mol Psychiatry.* 2014;19(12):1275–1283

55. National Scientific Council on the Developing Child. *Excessive Stress Disrupts the Architecture of the Developing Brain: Working Paper No. 3.* 2005/2014. https://developingchild.harvard.edu/resources/wp3. Accessed February 28, 2018

56. Tottenham N, Hare TA, Quinn BT, et al. Prolonged institutional rearing is associated with atypically large amygdala volume and difficulties in emotion regulation. *Dev Sci.* 2010;13(1):46–61

57. Lupien SJ, Parent S, Evans AC, et al. Larger amygdala but no change in hippocampal volume in 10-year-old children exposed to maternal depressive symptomatology since birth. *Proc Natl Acad Sci U S A.* 2011;108(34):14324–14329

58. Kim P, Evans GW, Angstadt M, et al. Effects of childhood poverty and chronic stress on emotion regulatory brain function in adulthood. *Proc Natl Acad Sci U S A.* 2013;110(46):18442–18447

59. Johnson SB, Riley AW, Granger DA, Riis J. The science of early life toxic stress for pediatric practice and advocacy. *Pediatrics.* 2013;131(2):319–327

Chapter 5

Thinking Developmentally

· ·

*"You never change things by fighting the existing reality.
To change something, build a new model that makes
the existing model obsolete."*

– R. Buckminster Fuller

· ·

For many pediatricians, "thinking developmentally" is intuitive. Cognitive frameworks used by pediatricians everyday include acknowledging the significant influences of the social milieu and past experiences on current behaviors; understanding the cumulative process of development and long-term consequences of early disruptions; recognizing that maladaptive behaviors are often maintained because they were actually adaptive at some point in the past; and generally thinking longitudinally over time. But for some health care professionals, unfamiliarity with recent advances in the basic developmental sciences, coupled with the time constraints of a busy clinical practice, limit consideration to the patient's current condition, often with little thought given to how they arrived at the current state or what that journey might mean for the future. This myopic vision not only is detrimental to patient care; it limits the way research is framed, trainees are instructed, and policy is crafted.

This chapter will briefly review the evolution of 3 models used to frame human health. This review is not intended to be comprehensive or all-inclusive because many other models of health have been proposed.[1–4] But many of their salient features align with one or more of the following 3 models: the biomedical (BM) model, the biopsychosocial (BPS) model, and

---

This chapter was originally published in slightly different form as Garner AS. Thinking developmentally: the next evolution in models of health. *J Dev Behav Pediatr.* 2016;37(7):579–584. Copyright 2016 Wolters Kluwer Health. Reprinted courtesy of Wolters Kluwer Health and the Society for Developmental and Behavioral Pediatrics.

the ecobiodevelopmental (EBD) model. By beginning with the BM model, the subsequent BPS and EBD models are understood as attempts to reconcile and integrate the BM model with subsequent advances in scientific knowledge, initially in the psychosocial sciences but more recently in the developmental sciences. In doing so, the BPS and EBD models not only redefine how to train for and practice medicine; they broaden the concept of "health" from simply the absence of disease to a dynamic spectrum that ranges from the presence of disease to the presence of wellness (Box 5-1).

Evolving Models of Disease, Health, and Wellness

Following advances in biology and other physical sciences at the end of the 19th century, much of Western medicine adopted a BM model of disease.[5] The BM model was grounded in biological reductionism, as advances in

Box 5-1. Evolving Models of Disease, Health, and Wellness

Biomedical Model of Disease (mid-19th century)
- Embraced biological reductionism (a single, organic etiology) and mind-body dualism (psychosocial vs organic etiologies; "problems of living" vs "problems of life").
- The practice of medicine demands an understanding of human biology and the physical sciences.
- Health is simply the absence of disease.

Biopsychosocial Model of Health (1977)
- Grounded in social-cognitive theory, refuted mind-body dualism, and embraced a broader vision of health.
- The practice of medicine demands an understanding of the nexus among human biology, psychology, and sociology.
- Health is the product of many factors and more than the absence of an objective disease state.

Ecobiodevelopmental Model of Disease and Wellness (2012)
- Driven by advances in basic developmental science (eg, epigenetics, developmental neuroscience), replaces mind-body dualism with adaptive versus maladaptive responses to experience, and acknowledges the developmental origins of disease and wellness.
- The practice of medicine demands an understanding of how the ecology (eg, the physical, nutritional, and psychosocial milieu) and biology (eg, genome, brain) interact in a dynamic and cumulative manner over time.
- Health is a dynamic continuum between disease and wellness, and early experiences play a pivotal role because the foundations for disease and wellness are built over time.

microbiology and Mendelian genetics suggested that one physical etiology (eg, a single germ, a single gene) could account for a diseased state. The BM also embraced a mind-body dualism, differentiating disorders of *living* (due to poor mental health, psychosocial circumstances, or poor character) from disorders of *life* (due to physical health and biology). The BM model of disease, therefore, demanded that health care professionals be well versed in human biology, including anatomy, physiology, histology, immunology, and microbiology. The vestiges of this BM model of disease are still seen in contemporary medical school curricula, with their emphasis on the physical sciences over the social sciences (eg, psychology, sociology, epidemiology, public health). According to the BM model, health is simply the absence of a diseased state.

In the 1970s, George Engel published a series papers outlining the need for a new medical model.[6-8] As a psychiatrist, Engel was steeped in social-cognitive theory and took exception to the concepts of biological reductionism and mind-body dualism. He argued that the BM model was "no longer adequate for the scientific tasks and social responsibilities of either medicine or psychiatry" because "it leaves no room within its framework for the social, psychological, and behavioral dimensions of disease."[8] As Engel stated, "We are now faced with the necessity and the challenge to broaden the approach to disease to include the psychosocial without sacrificing the enormous advantages of the biomedical approach."[8]

Engel proposed a BPS model that acknowledged the contributions of biology and physical science but also embraced the significant effect of nonorganic influences on health. The Engel BPS model presaged the contemporary appreciation for the social determinants of health and suggested that the practice of medicine demanded an understanding of the nexus among human biology, psychology, and sociology. In rejecting the extreme biological reductionism of the BM model, the BPS model embraced a systems approach (multifactorial etiologies) and suggested that health was more than the absence of a physical or objective diseased state.

In 2012, the American Academy of Pediatrics released a policy statement[9] and technical report[10] on toxic stress that endorsed an EBD model of disease and wellness. Integrating elements of several previous models, including the ecodevelopmental[3,11,12] and biodevelopmental[4] models, the EBD model affirms the BPS model's emphasis on the psychosocial determinants of health, but it does so at the molecular and cellular levels. According to the EBD model, the salient features of the early developmental milieu (ie, physical, nutritional, and psychosocial) are biologically embedded and influence the subsequent trajectory of development.[10] Recent advances in basic developmental sciences like epigenetics and neuroscience have begun to elucidate how the ecology gets under the skin[13,14] and influences genomic function, physiology, brain connectivity, learning, behavior, and, ultimately, life course trajectories (Figure 5-1).[2,15,16] Consequently, the EBD model argues that the practice of medicine requires an understanding of how the ecology and biology interact in a dynamic but cumulative manner over time. In the EBD model, health is a continuum between disease and wellness, and early experiences play a pivotal role because the foundations for both are built over time (see Box 5-1).

Advantages of the Ecobiodevelopmental Model

The EBD model builds and improves on the BM and BPS models. Like the BM model, the EBD model is grounded in contemporary basic science (eg, epigenetics, neuroscience). Like the BPS model, the EBD model affirms the biological significance of the salient features of the ecology, including

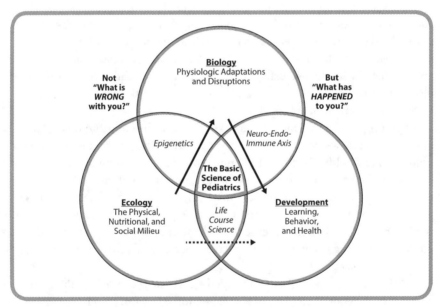

Figure 5-1. The emerging model of how the ecology affects development. Life course science has repeatedly demonstrated strong associations (dotted arrow) between the early childhood ecology and developmental outcomes in learning, behavior, and health. Through epigenetic mechanisms (solid arrow), the early childhood ecology is biologically embedded, leading to changes in the way the genetic blueprint is used. Developmental neuroscience helps us to understand how those biological changes (adaptive and disruptive) lead to alterations in brain structure and function. But the biological changes in response to the environment extend beyond the nervous system and include alterations to endocrine and immune function as well. Adaptive and disruptive changes in this neuro-endo-immune axis drive lifelong outcomes in learning, behavior, and health (solid arrow). In the center of this Venn diagram is what Dr Julius Richmond called the "basic science of pediatrics": the basic science of child development. One important implication of this emerging model is that asking patients, "What is wrong with you?" is not as salient as asking, "What has happened to you?"

the psychosocial milieu. What sets the EBD model apart is that it adds the dimension of time, forcing health care professionals to think developmentally (Figure 5-2).

The EBD model acknowledges that development is the product of an ongoing, dynamic, but cumulative dance between nurture (the environmental milieu or ecology) and nature (biology).[9,17] The advances in epigenetics and developmental neuroscience discussed in the previous 2 chapters demonstrate that experiences with the physical, nutritional, and psychosocial ecology lead to changes in genomic function, physiology, and brain connectivity.[16] At the highest level, the output of all of these ecologically induced changes is behavior, which, in turn, shapes the individual's next experience with the ecology. This ongoing and dynamic dance between ecology and biology is depicted in Figure 5-2A.

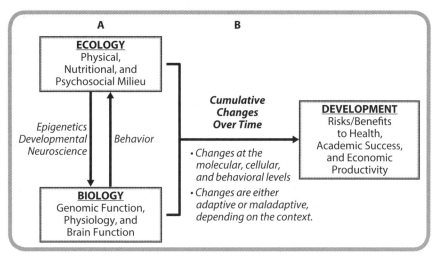

Figure 5-2. The ecobiodevelopmental (EBD) model of disease and wellness. The ecology becomes biology, and together they drive the development of disease and wellness across the life span.
A. There is an ongoing, dynamic dance between the ecology and biology. The biomedical model focused primarily on the biology. The biopsychosocial model acknowledged the psychosocial components of the ecology, but recent advances in epigenetics and developmental neuroscience have revealed molecular and cellular mechanisms that allow the ecology to become biologically embedded. Conversely, the highest-level output of biology is behavior, which shapes the individual's next experience with the ecology.
B. Cumulative changes over time drive development and lead to risks and benefits to health, academic success, and economic productivity. The dynamic dance between the ecology and biology lead to changes at the molecular (eg, DNA methylation), cellular (eg, brain connectivity), and behavioral levels (eg, behavioral allostasis). Although these changes might be adaptive initially (eg, the physiologic stress response), they might prove to be maladaptive over time (eg, toxic stress) or in different contexts (eg, post-traumatic stress). The EBD model adds this dimension of time and forces health care professionals to think developmentally.

The EBD model asserts that, over time, the accumulation of changes at the molecular, cellular, and behavioral levels in response to the ecology can be adaptive or maladaptive, depending on the subsequent context (Figure 5-2B). For example, significant adversity early in life can lead to changes in methylation patterns (eg, the glucocorticoid receptor gene),[18] brain connectivity (eg, a reduced capacity for the prefrontal cortex to suppress the amygdala),[19] and coping behaviors (eg, behavioral allostasis manifest as smoking, overeating, promiscuity, or substance abuse)[20,21] that might be somewhat adaptive and beneficial initially but prove to be maladaptive or harmful over time. These adaptive and maladaptive changes due to the ecology represent benefits and risks to not only health but academic success and future economic productivity (see Figure 5-2).[10]

The EBD model also

1. Eliminates mind-body dualism. The dichotomy of disorders of *living* versus disorders of *life* is replaced with the dichotomy of *adaptive* versus *maladaptive* changes at the molecular, cellular, and behavioral levels in response to experiences with the ecology. Those changes caused by the psychosocial features of the ecology are, therefore, every bit as biological as the changes caused by physiological factors such as poor nutrition or lead poisoning.

2. Incorporates potentially transformational advances in epigenetics and developmental neuroscience. Plasticity, the ability of genomic and brain function to be altered by experiences with the ecology, is a powerful resource, but it cuts both ways. Early experiences can set a strong or weak foundation for future learning, health, and economic success.[22]

3. Is congruent with the burgeoning literature on gene and environmental interactions,[23] including intriguing evidence that a biological sensitivity to context can be a benefit in nurturing environments but a risk in adverse environments.[24–29]

4. Highlights the pivotal role of the early childhood ecology. In the absence of safe, stable, and nurturing relationships, significant adversity in childhood can lead to toxic stress responses. Frequent, prolonged, or overexposure to the mediators of the physiologic stress response triggers changes at the molecular, cellular, and behavioral levels that may prove to be unhealthy over time. Conversely, the presence of safe, stable, and nurturing relationships (with parents, caregivers, extended family, teachers, and coaches) buffers adversity, triggering a positive stress response that is infrequent or brief, leads to healthy adaptations to future adversity, and builds competence and confidence. Significant adversity in childhood can indeed be toxic, but safe, stable, and nurturing relationships are the antidote.[30]

5. Incorporates recent epidemiologic studies that suggest many chronic diseases are actually adult-*manifest* diseases with origins in childhood. The Adverse Childhood Experiences (ACE) Study,[20,21] the data supporting the so-called Barker or fetal origins hypothesis,[31,32] and the burgeoning field of study loosely referred to as the developmental origins of health and disease[33–36] all force health care professionals to begin considering distal or remote etiologies. The history of the ACE Study is a cautionary tale for non-pediatric health care professionals, as an internist discovered that significant adversity in childhood was preventing many of his adult patients who were morbidly obese from maintaining their weight loss.[21] By understanding the remote or distal causes of maladaptations, and by uncovering the adversities that may have led to behavioral allostasis, health care professionals are in a better position to form strong therapeutic relationships, empower patients with a deeper understanding as to why they may feel stuck in unhealthy behaviors, and support patients in developing ways first to heal and then to cope more adaptively moving forward. With regard to this last point and the need to build wellness moving forward, motivational interviewing and cognitive behavioral strategies may prove useful.

6. Forces health care professionals to think developmentally. Although trauma-informed care also encourages health care professionals to change their approach from "What is wrong with you?" to "What has happened to you?"[37] an emphasis on the *risks* to health must be balanced with the *benefits* to health that come from strong social supports (eg, family), mindfulness (eg, emotional intelligence), healthy adaptations to previous adversity (eg, exercise, journaling, artistic pursuits), and other sources of resilience. The EBD model embraces reactive, trauma-informed care *and* proactive, resilience-informed care under the broader umbrella of development-informed care.

7. Challenges the medical community to accept a broader vision and mission, because thinking developmentally demands that one also think ecologically. As discussed earlier in this chapter, the accumulation of changes due to experiences with the environment shapes who we are at the molecular, cellular, and behavioral levels. To address the biology underlying disparities and to optimize adult outcomes, not just in health but in academic achievement and economic productivity, medicine must accept an expanded vision that acknowledges the social determinants of health and the developmental origins of disease and wellness. The mission, therefore, expands from "How do we cure the sick?" to include "How do we build the well?"

Implications for the Health Care System

Meeting this expanded mission and vision will demand dramatic changes in the health care system. The EBD model's emphasis on the development of wellness was mirrored in the efforts of the original Patient Protection and Affordable Care Act (ACA) to support prevention services. Similarly, the EBD model's emphasis on optimizing the ecology was mirrored in the focus of the original ACA on measuring and improving population-level health. But change is hard, and skeptics will continue to argue that the social determinants of health and other factors of the ecology that build disease instead of wellness are beyond the scope of medicine. Yet even the skeptics will concede that, while our current system is well prepared to cure the sick, the system is simply unsustainable economically. In addition, our overall health, by any number of measures, is poor relative to our economic peers.[38] For every dollar that economically advanced countries spend on medical care, they spend 2 dollars on the social services that promote healthy ecologies.[39] In the United States, for every dollar we spend on medical care, we spend 90 cents on social services.[39] The EBD model predicts that the way to build wellness and to decrease health care expenditures over the long term is to promote healthier ecologies.[10]

But this dichotomy between social services and medical expenditures is grounded in mind-body dualism and the artificial dichotomy between disorders of *living* and disorders of *life*. From an economic standpoint, investments in social services and health care are complementary investments in human capital. That is not to say that physicians are now social workers, but that physicians and social workers are now working toward the same end: child, family, and community wellness. The same could be said for early intervention specialists, home visitors, legal advocates, educators, and job-training professionals. The EBD model supports the concept of community-based, family-centered medical homes, where a team of professionals is led by a physician and focuses not only on curing the sick but on building the well.

For many health care centers, however, this transition from curing the sick to building the well will require a significant redistribution of resources. Does the community need more medical specialists or more home visitors and community health workers? Does the community need another magnetic resonance imaging scanner or another well-located primary care clinic? More importantly, this transition to a well-care system will require a fundamental shift in the relationship between tertiary care centers and primary care physicians. In the sick-care system, one of the principal roles of primary care physicians is to feed the centers with sick patients in need of high-tech, expensive, tertiary care. In a well-care system, tertiary care centers must empower primary care physicians with the tools needed to improve the lives of children, their families, and their communities. Resources like community health workers, home visiting programs,[30] medicolegal partnerships,[40] and Health Leads[41] allow academic health care centers to begin changing the directionality from "feed us the sick" to "let us help you keep people well" outside the tertiary care center.

If changing this directionality sounds naive, consider the example of episode-based payments for asthma. Under this model, if a child presents to the emergency department of a tertiary care center with an asthma exacerbation, the tertiary care center payment for that visit may cover the patient's asthma care for the next 30 days. If, after discharge, the patient is subsequently readmitted to the intensive care unit during those next 30 days, the tertiary care center would get no additional payment. Hence, tertiary care centers are now incentivized to ensure compliance with the treatment plan and adequate follow-up with the primary care physician. But the primary care physician will likely point out that to prevent readmissions, a home visit is needed to ensure that the home space is being adequately maintained by the landlord (eg, absence of mold or cockroaches). If it is not, the family may need the assistance of a medicolegal partnership to minimize the risk of a subsequent readmission. This example demonstrates the need for tertiary care centers to seek bidirectionality in their relationships with primary care physicians and the communities they serve. To promote wellness, health care centers need to carefully consider ways to assist primary care physicians and other local resources (eg, food pantries, domestic violence or homeless shelters, Head Start, neighborhood resource centers) in keeping children, their families, and their communities well.

Implications for Medical Practice and Training

Transitioning to a well-care system will also require changes in the way that physicians practice medicine. As described in the EBD model, physicians must begin to think developmentally and ecologically. Thinking developmentally forces physicians to acknowledge the significant biological consequences of previous experiences, both good and bad. When thinking developmentally, the most important question for physicians to consider is not "What is *wrong* with this patient?" but "What has *happened* to this patient?"[37] When thinking developmentally, physicians will be challenged to ask themselves, "How can I *better understand* this patient?" instead of "How can I *fix* this patient?" Thinking developmentally acknowledges that the patient's current health status is the product of their previous experiences. Thinking developmentally encourages physicians to "go upstream" and consider the distal or remote etiologies (eg, the link between significant adversity in childhood and adult obesity). But to assess the patient's history and ecology in a safe, nonjudg-mental, and respectful manner, physicians must redouble their efforts to form therapeutic relationships and to always be mindful of their own vicarious trauma on hearing the patient's experiences. If the physician's orientation is, "I must fix this," they are likely to face rising levels of frustration and burnout. But if the physician's orientation is, "I must understand this patient," they are more likely to practice active listening, form that foundational therapeutic relationship, and protect themselves from the frustration of not being able to fix the patient's experience.

The EBD model will also challenge physicians to think ecologically, not only about etiologies but also interventions and treatments. Thinking ecologically will encourage physicians to adopt a public health approach to complex issues (eg, obesity) and to capitalize on individual, family, and community strengths and assets. For example, if a child has an identified learning disability, efforts might be made to strengthen that child's social-emotional skills to empower the child to successfully engage assistance when needed. If a family is strug-gling due to maternal depression, efforts might be made to garner additional supports from the extended family or a faith community. Similarly, communi-ties could work to ensure that although its children may live in poverty, they will not be impoverished socially, emotionally, or intellectually.

To prepare the next generation of health care professionals for this emerg-ing well-care system, undergraduate medical education will need to embrace the EBD model of disease and wellness. All physicians will need to start thinking developmentally and ecologically. As the leaders of teams of health care professionals, the next generation of physicians must also develop the skills needed to collaborate with a wide range of professionals outside the tra-ditional purview of medicine. Perhaps most importantly, to prepare the next generation of pediatricians, pediatric residency programs will need to expand the time allotted for developmental and behavioral pediatrics, both to reassert that child development is the basic science of pediatrics[42] and to operational-ize the broad implications of the EBD model.

Conclusions From Part 1

To transition from a health care system that reactively cures the sick to one that proactively builds the well, a different model of health is needed. The EBD model of disease and wellness is grounded in contemporary advances in devel-opmental science (chapters 1–4), builds on previous models of health (Chapter 5), eliminates mind-body dualism (the idea that mental health and physical health are somehow distinct), and challenges health care professionals to think developmentally. Thinking developmentally acknowledges the ongoing but cumulative dance over time between the salient features of the ecology and the biological machinery that is adapting, for better or worse, to that ecology. Thinking developmentally also means thinking ecologically because the accumulation of experiences with the environment shapes who we are at the molecular, cellular, and behavioral levels.

Part 2 of this book will build on these foundational principles and expand the discussion of the implications of the EBD model to children (Chapter 6), their families (Chapter 7), their communities (Chapter 8), the future practice of pediatrics (Chapter 9), and public policy (Chapter 10). The emerging developmental science discussed in this and the previous 4 chapters is solid. The question to be addressed in the second half of this book is what we, as pediatricians, parents, and citizens, can do to translate this emerging science into healthy children, nurturing families, and caring communities. As pediatricians, that's what we do: translate the latest science into practice and policy. That has been, and hopefully will remain, the pediatric way.

References

1. Halfon N, Hochstein M. Life course health development: an integrated framework for developing health, policy, and research. *Milbank Q.* 2002;80(3):433–479
2. Hertzman C, Power C. Health and human development: understandings from life-course research. *Dev Neuropsychol.* 2003;24(2-3):719–744
3. Bronfenbrenner U, ed. *Making Human Beings Human: Bioecological Perspectives on Human Development.* Thousand Oaks, CA: Sage Publications; 2005
4. Shonkoff JP. Building a new biodevelopmental framework to guide the future of early childhood policy. *Child Dev.* 2010;81(1):357–367
5. Annandale E. *The Sociology of Health and Medicine: A Critical Introduction.* 2nd ed. Malden, MA: Polity Press; 2014
6. Engel GL. The biopsychosocial model and the education of health professionals. *Gen Hosp Psychiatry.* 1979;1(2):156–165
7. Engel GL. The biopsychosocial model and the education of health professionals. *Ann N Y Acad Sci.* 1978;310:169–187
8. Engel GL. The need for a new medical model: a challenge for biomedicine. *Science.* 1977;196(4286):129–136
9. American Academy of Pediatrics Committee on Psychosocial Aspects of Child and Family Health; Committee on Early Childhood, Adoption, and Dependent Care; Section on Developmental and Behavioral Pediatrics. Policy statement: early childhood adversity, toxic stress, and the role of the pediatrician: translating developmental science into lifelong health. *Pediatrics.* 2012;129(1):e224–e231
10. Shonkoff JP, Garner AS; American Academy of Pediatrics Committee on Psychosocial Aspects of Child and Family Health; Committee on Early Childhood, Adoption, and Dependent Care; Section on Developmental and Behavioral Pediatrics. Technical report: the lifelong effects of early childhood adversity and toxic stress. *Pediatrics.* 2012;129(1):e232–e246
11. Moen P, Elder GH, Lüscher K, eds. *Examining Lives in Context: Perspectives on the Ecology of Human Development.* Washington, DC: American Psychological Association; 1995

12. Bronfenbrenner U. *The Ecology of Human Development: Experiments by Nature and Design.* Cambridge, MA: Harvard University Press; 1979

13. Hertzman C. The biological embedding of early experience and its effects on health in adulthood. *Ann N Y Acad Sci.* 1999;896:85–95

14. Hertzman C, Boyce T. How experience gets under the skin to create gradients in developmental health. *Annu Rev Public Health.* 2010;31:329–347

15. Royal Society of Canada and the Canadian Academy of Health Sciences. *Early Child Development: Adverse Experiences and Developmental Health.* Ottawa, ON: Royal Society of Canada; 2012

16. Shonkoff JP, Boyce WT, McEwen BS. Neuroscience, molecular biology, and the childhood roots of health disparities: building a new framework for health promotion and disease prevention. *JAMA.* 2009;301(21):2252–2259

17. Hertzman C, Power C, Matthews S, Manor O. Using an interactive framework of society and lifecourse to explain self-rated health in early adulthood. *Soc Sci Med.* 2001;53(12):1575–1585

18. Oberlander TF, Weinberg J, Papsdorf M, Grunau R, Misri S, Devlin AM. Prenatal exposure to maternal depression, neonatal methylation of human glucocorticoid receptor gene (NR3C1) and infant cortisol stress responses. *Epigenetics.* 2008;3(2):97–106

19. Kim P, Evans GW, Angstadt M, et al. Effects of childhood poverty and chronic stress on emotion regulatory brain function in adulthood. *Proc Natl Acad Sci U S A.* 2013;110(46):18442–18447

20. Anda RF, Felitti VJ, Bremner JD, et al. The enduring effects of abuse and related adverse experiences in childhood. A convergence of evidence from neurobiology and epidemiology. *Eur Arch Psychiatry Clin Neurosci.* 2006;256(3):174–186

21. Felitti VJ, Anda RF, Nordenberg D, et al. Relationship of childhood abuse and household dysfunction to many of the leading causes of death in adults. The Adverse Childhood Experiences (ACE) Study. *Am J Prev Med.* 1998;14(4):245–258

22. National Research Council, Institute of Medicine. *From Neurons to Neighborhoods: The Science of Early Child Development.* Committee on Integrating the Science of Early Childhood Development. Shonkoff JP, Phillips DA, eds. Washington, DC: National Academy Press; 2000

23. Simons RL, Beach SR, Barr AB. Differential susceptibility to context: a promising model of the interplay of genes and the social environment. *Adv Group Process.* 2012;29

24. Ellis BJ, Essex MJ, Boyce WT. Biological sensitivity to context: II. Empirical explorations of an evolutionary-developmental theory. *Dev Psychopathol.* 2005;17(2):303–328

25. Boyce WT, Ellis BJ. Biological sensitivity to context: I. An evolutionary-developmental theory of the origins and functions of stress reactivity. *Dev Psychopathol.* 2005;17(2):271–301

26. Obradović J, Bush NR, Stamperdahl J, Adler NE, Boyce WT. Biological sensitivity to context: the interactive effects of stress reactivity and family adversity on socioemotional behavior and school readiness. *Child Dev.* 2010;81(1):270–289

27. Obradović J, Boyce WT. Individual differences in behavioral, physiological, and genetic sensitivities to contexts: implications for development and adaptation. *Dev Neurosci.* 2009;31(4):300–308

28. Blair C, Raver CC. Child development in the context of adversity: experiential canalization of brain and behavior. *Am Psychol.* 2012;67(4):309–318

29. Blair C. Stress and the development of self-regulation in context. *Child Dev Perspect.* 2010;4(3):181–188

30. Garner AS. Home visiting and the biology of toxic stress: opportunities to address early childhood adversity. *Pediatrics.* 2013;132(Suppl 2):S65–S73

31. Barker DJ. Fetal origins of cardiovascular disease. *Ann Med.* 1999;31(Suppl 1):3–6

32. Barker DJ. Fetal origins of coronary heart disease. *BMJ.* 1995;311(6998):171–174

33. Barker D, Barker M, Fleming T, Lampl M. Developmental biology: support mothers to secure future public health. *Nature.* 2013;504(7479):209–211

34. Barker DJ. The origins of the developmental origins theory. *J Intern Med.* 2007;261(5): 412–417

35. Gluckman PD, Hanson MA, Buklijas T. A conceptual framework for the developmental origins of health and disease. *J Dev Orig Health Dis.* 2010;1(1):6–18

36. Walker CL, Ho SM. Developmental reprogramming of cancer susceptibility. *Nat Rev Cancer.* 2012;12(7):479–486

37. Bloom SL. The sanctuary model: developing generic inpatient programs for the treatment of psychological trauma. In: Williams MB, Sommer JF, eds. *Handbook of Post-Traumatic Therapy.* Westport, CT: Greenwood Publishing; 1994:474–449

38. National Research Council, Institute of Medicine. *US Health in International Perspective: Shorter Lives, Poorer Health.* Washington, DC: National Academies Press; 2013

39. Bradley EH, Elkins BR, Herrin J, Elbel B. Health and social services expenditures: associations with health outcomes. *BMJ Qual Saf.* 2011;20(10):826–831

40. Sege R, Preer G, Morton SJ, et al. Medical-legal strategies to improve infant health care: a randomized trial. *Pediatrics.* 2015;136(1):97–106

41. Onie RD. Creating a new model to help health care providers write prescriptions for health. *Health Aff (Millwood).* 2012;31(12):2795–2796

42. Richmond JB. Child development: a basic science for pediatrics. *Pediatrics.* 1967;39(5): 649–658

Part 2: Translating Developmental Science Into Practice and Policy

Chapter 6

The Biological Needs of Young Children

• •

In the 13th century, the Holy Roman Emperor Frederick II "...wanted to find out what kind of speech and what manner of speech children would have when they grew up, if they spoke to no one beforehand. So he bade foster mothers and nurses to suckle the children, to bathe and wash them, but in no way to prattle with them or to speak to them...But he laboured in vain, because the children all died. For they could not live without the petting and the joyful faces and loving words of their foster mothers."

– Salimbene (13th-century Franciscan)[1,2]

• •

Part 1 discusses the recent advances in developmental science that underlie the ecobiodevelopmental (EBD) model and highlights the inadequacies of previous models of health. In the second half of this book, we will explore the implications of these advances and the EBD model for parenting, practicing medicine, and formulating public policy. The contemporary challenge facing health care professionals, educators, child advocates, policy makers, and parents is to translate the science of early child development into practices and policies that yield healthier children today and healthier life course trajectories for the engaged, productive citizens of the future. How do we collectively nurture wellness in childhood to promote lifelong health?

No Magic Bullet

As discussed in the previous chapter, the EBD model should facilitate this process by providing a perspective that is unique to pediatrics—one that thinks developmentally and focuses on the early childhood ecology. Through this lens, it quickly becomes apparent that within any given child's ecology, there are innumerable potential precipitants of toxic stress that could become impediments to optimal development. The EBD model, therefore, suggests that there will be no single, magic bullet intervention that addresses all these potential impediments, nor one that simultaneously prevents, mitigates, and treats childhood adversity. Toxic stress is best addressed by way of a public health approach (Figure 6-1), with layered or nested programs that not only heal the sick but proactively build the well. Such an approach will need to include

1. Tangible, universal, primary preventions *for all children* that build the rudiments of resilience in preparation for future adversity
2. Cost-effective, targeted interventions *for children at risk* for significant adversity
3. Accessible, evidence-based treatments *for children who are already experiencing toxic stress* in response to adversity

To successfully address early childhood adversity and toxic stress and to measurably promote childhood wellness and healthy life course trajectories, efforts will need to be made at all 3 of these public health levels. This has been referred to as *vertical integration* (see Figure 6-1), whereas *horizontal integration* refers to efforts that include not only health care but the educational, social service, and juvenile justice systems.[3]

The EBD model predicts that to improve developmental outcomes and life course trajectories, efforts must be made to improve the early childhood ecology. Unmet needs in early childhood are among the potential precipitants of toxic stress responses. This chapter will explore what the most basic biological needs of young children are, as well as what can and should be done to meet those most basic needs. Parents have similar basic needs, so this chapter will also introduce the concept of 2-generation approaches, but a more detailed discussion of parental needs will be reserved for the next chapter. Finally, this chapter will highlight the need to understand social contexts and the so-called social determinants of health in order to apply the basic science tenets of Part 1 to the interventions and policy strategies discussed here and throughout the rest of the book.

Stepping on the Gas Versus Releasing the Brake

When childhood adversity triggers a toxic stress response, changes in the genome and brain architecture may initially be adaptive, but they prove to

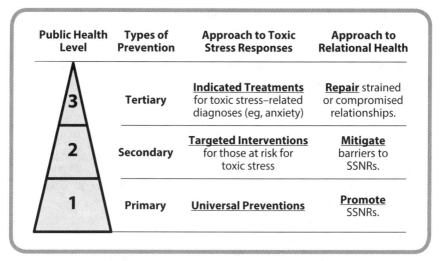

Figure 6-1. A public health approach includes 1) universal, primary preventions; 2) targeted interventions for those at higher risk (secondary prevention); and 3) indicated treatments for those with diagnoses to prevent the progression of disease (tertiary prevention). Given that safe, stable, and nurturing relationships (SSNRs) are the antidote to toxic stress, an analogous approach based on relational health would include efforts that 1) proactively promote SSNRs, 2) mitigate barriers to SSNRs, and 3) repair relationships that are strained or compromised. Public health approaches that are *vertically integrated* include elements of all 3 levels. Public health approaches that are *horizontally integrated* cut across silos and include not only health care but the educational, social service, and juvenile justice systems.[3]

be maladaptive over time or in different contexts. For example, if a child's amygdala becomes larger or more potent in response to childhood neglect, maternal depression, or poverty, that may prepare the young child for a dog-eat-dog world.[4–7] But the amygdala is also capable of inhibiting the activity of the hippocampus and prefrontal cortex, 2 areas known to be important for learning and adaptive behaviors.[8,9]

This discovery has profound implications for education and learning. Much of our educational system is based on the idea that we (parents, teachers, and society as a whole) must step on the gas by stimulating children and drilling them to practice and eventually master new skills. But the emerging biological model is that we must first release the brake by preventing and mitigating the toxic stress responses that inhibit optimal early brain and child development. The recent advances in developmental biology discussed in Part 1 suggest that protecting the brain from toxic stress will release a potent brake on the brain's development, allowing the forming brain to be more receptive to those stimulating educational experiences.[10]

In reality, of course, the educational model of stepping on the gas and the biological model of releasing the brake are 2 sides of the same coin—the yin and yang of early childhood. Protecting the brain releases the brake of toxic stress and allows children to build new skills. But when building new skills, we should prioritize those skills that will decrease future toxic stress and continue to protect the brain (ie, foundational social, emotional, language, and adaptive skills) (Figure 6-2).

In fact, releasing potential brakes on or inhibitors of early brain and child development is not a new idea at all. At the dawn of the 20th century, Maria Montessori, Italy's first female pediatrician, was assigned to care for children with significant delays in development. She noted that these children demonstrated an innate drive to master new skills. Even if it was simply dropping a pencil over and over again, the child would do it until that new skill was

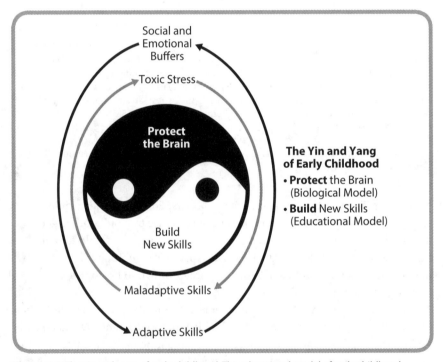

Figure 6-2. The yin and yang of early childhood. The educational model of early childhood learning is to step on the gas and build new skills by stimulating and repetitively drilling children. The emerging biological model is to release the brake and protect the brain by preventing and mitigating early childhood adversity and toxic stress. Because toxic stress negatively affects the functioning of the prefrontal cortex and hippocampus, early childhood adversity makes it harder for young children to learn new skills and adaptive behaviors (eg, understanding and regulating their emotions) and more likely that they will develop maladaptive behaviors (eg, withdrawal, aggression). These maladaptive behaviors lead to social isolation and more toxic stress over time (gray arrows). In the presence of social and emotional buffers (safe, stable, and nurturing relationships), the brake is released and children are better positioned to learn the new skills and adaptive behaviors that engender more social and emotional supports over time (black arrows).

mastered; then the child would move on to mastering another skill. When she also observed this innate drive to master in typical children, it became a lynchpin in her educational method.[11,12] Montessori explained, "We discovered that education is not something which the teacher does, but that it is a natural process which develops spontaneously in the human being."[13] Hence, the role of parents and teachers is to release any potential brakes that might inhibit that process, to order or arrange the environment so that the natural, spontaneous process of child development simply unfolds in an unimpeded manner. This breakthrough presaged the EBD model's emphasis on getting the ecology right to improve developmental outcomes.

The Concept of Self-actualization

In 1939, Kurt Goldstein described *self-actualization* as the internal drive to realize one's capabilities.[14] Fifteen years later, Abraham Maslow incorporated self-actualization into his theory of motivation and his hierarchy of needs.[15] According to Maslow, individuals are intrinsically motivated to meet 2 different types of needs: *deficiency needs* and *growth needs.* Deficiency needs include physiologic needs (eg, food, water, sleep); the need to feel safe; the need to feel understood by and connected to others; and the need to feel competent and to maintain one's self-esteem. Maslow concluded that meeting these deficiency needs allowed some individuals to experience *meta-motivation,* or the intrinsic drive to meet growth needs, like self-actualization and transcendence (Box 6-1).[16] Conversely, when the deficiency needs are not met, self-actualization and transcendence are made more difficult, if not impossible. Although many parents would be content if their children were to become self-actualizers, in Maslow's later writings, he argued that our ultimate meta-motivation is toward transcendence and the acknowledgment of realities beyond one's self (ie, altruism, an appreciation of beauty, or an awareness of one's spirituality).[16] Maslow argued that meeting a person's deficiency needs unmasks their innate meta-motivation to self-actualize and possibly even to transcend their own experience.

Like Montessori, Maslow presaged the recent advances in developmental science and the realization that optimal child development depends on the ability of the childhood milieu to release an intrinsic drive to master. He wrote, "All the evidence that we have indicates that it is reasonable to assume in practically every human being, and certainly in almost every newborn baby, that there is an active will toward health, an impulse towards growth, or towards the actualization."[17] But when needs such as food, safety, and connectedness are left unmet, they become barriers to self-actualization. Today we recognize these so-called social determinants of health as precipitants of toxic stress and barriers to optimal early brain and child development.

Box 6-1. Maslow Hierarchy of Needs and Motivations

DEFICIENCY NEEDS AND SOURCES OF MOTIVATION

1. Physiologic Needs
   - Basic metabolic requirements
     ◦ Air
     ◦ Food
     ◦ Water
   - Clothing
   - Shelter
2. Safety Needs
   - Personal security
   - Financial security
   - Health and well-being
   - Safety net against accidents and illness
3. Love and Belonging (Connectivity)
   - Friendship
   - Intimacy
   - Family
4. Self-esteem (Competencies and a Sense of Agency)
   - Valued by others
   - Self-respect

GROWTH NEEDS AND SOURCES OF META-MOTIVATION

5. Self-actualization (being true to oneself)
   - Utilizing one's capabilities
   - Fulfilling one's potential
6. Transcendence (moving beyond oneself)
   - Altruism
   - Spirituality

Applying Maslow's Theory to Today's Children and Parents

Maslow's concepts of deficiency needs and self-actualization provide a framework for considering the needs and goals of contemporary children and their parents (Table 6-1). For example, if our measure of self-actualization is children coming to school ready, willing, and able to learn, Maslow would argue that they would first need to have their deficiency needs met. If children are hungry or do not get enough sleep (their physiologic needs), it might be hard for them to come to school ready to learn. If their safety needs are not met because they are preoccupied with the bullies on the bus, they might not be ready to learn. If their need for connection or love is not met because no single teacher in the school believes in them, shows them affection, or even notices if they are there or not there from one day to the next, they might not be ready

Table 6-1. Applying Maslow's Theory to Today's Children and Parents Reveals Deficiency Needs as Potential Barriers to Self-actualization

	Today's Children	Today's Parents
When Needs Are Met (Self-actualization)	Children go to school ready and willing to learn.	Parents are the best versions of themselves.
When Needs Are Not Met (Deficiency Needs)	Children are not ready and/or motivated to learn.	Parents cannot be the types of parents they wish to be.
Self-esteem Deficiency	No chance to excel (eg, no sports, music, art)	No chance to contribute (eg, no job)
Love/Connection Deficiency	No bonds with teachers	No community supports
Safety Deficiency	Bullies on the bus	Domestic violence
Biological Deficiency	Hungry or poor sleep	Food or housing insecurity

to learn. Or, if they are not gifted cognitively but they excel in sports, music, or the visual arts, but their deficiency need for esteem and recognition is not met because the district just cut athletic activities, music class, and art, they might not be fully ready or motivated to learn. According to Maslow's theory, if we want our children to be self-motivated learners and to come to school ready, willing, and able to learn, we need to ensure that their deficiency needs—their most basic biological needs—are met.

But consider for a moment the barriers preventing parents from being the best possible versions of themselves or from becoming the type of parents they most wish to be. As pediatricians with more than a half-century's worth of combined professional experience, we will attest that the vast majority of parents genuinely want to do right by their children. But Maslow's theory would suggest that if the parents' own physiologic needs are not met because of food insecurity or homelessness, it might be considerably harder for them to be the best possible versions of themselves. Likewise, if their safety needs are not met because of domestic violence; if their need for connection or love is not met because they have no spouse, extended family, or community supports; or if their esteem needs are not met because they have been left unemployed, they may not be the best possible versions of themselves. According to Maslow's theory, if we want parents to be the engaged mothers and fathers they already long to be, we must adopt a 2-generation perspective that also strives to meet the deficiency needs of the parents. We will return to and expand on this concept of helping the parents to help the children in the next chapter.

Empiric Data From America's Promise Alliance

Unmet needs are potential precipitants of toxic stress responses for children and their parents, and Maslow's theory is entirely congruent with the recent advances in developmental science. But Maslow's theory is just that—a theory. What empiric data do we have that these deficiency needs—these most basic biological needs—are barriers to long-term well-being and success?

Briefly consider the important work of America's Promise Alliance. To improve high school graduation rates, they have argued that children must have 5 "promises" met: a healthy start; safe places to live, learn, and play; caring adults and family; opportunities to contribute; and an effective education.[18] If these promises sound familiar, consider how they compare to Maslow's first 5 levels of needs (Table 6-2).

Although Maslow's levels of needs make sense intuitively, the 5 promises provide an evidence base. A 2006 report from America's Promise Alliance, *Every Child, Every Promise: Turning Failure Into Action,* provides extensive data about benefits of individuals living in an environment that fulfills many of the promises (Figure 6-3). The research found that "children who enjoy the

Table 6-2. Comparison of Maslow's 5 Levels of Needs With America's Promise Alliance 5 Promises

Needs	Models	
	Maslow's Hierarchy of Needs (Theoretical, 1943)	America's Promise Alliance (Evidence Based)
Self-actualization	Need to know, explore, and understand	An effective education
Esteem	Need to achieve and be recognized	Opportunities to contribute
Love/connection	Need for friends and social connections	Caring adults and family
Safety/security	Need to feel secure and safe from danger	Safe places to live, learn, and play
Physiologic	Need to satisfy hunger, thirst, and sleep	A healthy start

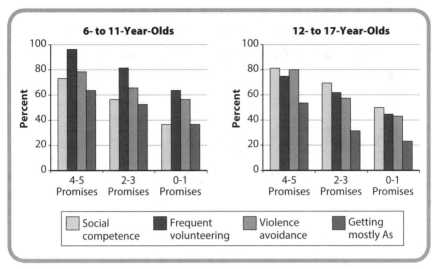

Figure 6-3. Children who experience at least 4 of the 5 promises are significantly more likely to be successful, measured by 4 indicators: social competence, frequent volunteering, violence avoidance, and getting mostly As.

From America's Promise Alliance. *Every Child, Every Promise: Turning Failure Into Action.* Washington, DC: America's Promise Alliance; 2006. http://www.americaspromise.org/sites/default/files/d8/Every%20Child%20Every%20Promise%20-%20Full%20Report.pdf. Accessed February 28, 2018.

sustained and cumulative benefit of having at least four of the Five Promises across various contexts of their lives are much more likely to be academically successful, civically engaged and socially competent, *regardless of their race or family income*"[18] (emphasis added).

Consider the significance of that last statement. Pediatricians, policy makers, child advocates, and parents have long decried racial and socioeconomic disparities in health, academic achievement, and economic productivity. Evidence from the America's Promise Alliance suggests that these disparities, these social or societal determinants of health, education, and welfare, can be mitigated or even eliminated by ensuring that all children have these 5 promises met.

The problem is that fewer than 1 in 3 children in the United States have 4 or 5 of the promises kept (Figure 6-4). Worse yet, about 1 in 5 children in the United States have none or only one of the promises kept. Additional information on unkept promises is found in Box 6-2. These statistics demonstrate that, for an untenable proportion of America's children, a tremendous amount of work is yet to be done to address deficits in equal opportunity. Too many children do not have a fair chance at self-actualization due to unmet deficiency needs, early childhood adversity, and toxic stress.

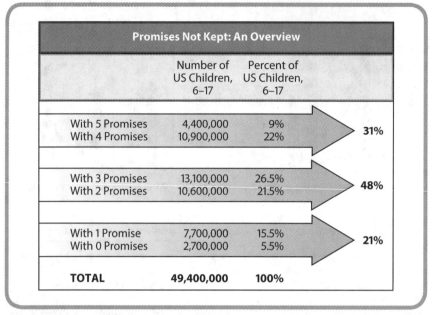

Promises Not Kept: An Overview		
	Number of US Children, 6–17	Percent of US Children, 6–17
With 5 Promises	4,400,000	9%
With 4 Promises	10,900,000	22%
With 3 Promises	13,100,000	26.5%
With 2 Promises	10,600,000	21.5%
With 1 Promise	7,700,000	15.5%
With 0 Promises	2,700,000	5.5%
TOTAL	**49,400,000**	**100%**

(Arrows: With 5 & 4 Promises → 31%; With 3 & 2 Promises → 48%; With 1 & 0 Promises → 21%)

Figure 6-4. Unkept promises and America's children.
From America's Promise Alliance. *Every Child, Every Promise: Turning Failure Into Action.* Washington, DC: America's Promise Alliance; 2006. http://www.americaspromise.org/sites/default/files/d8/Every%20Child%20Every%20Promise%20-%20Full%20Report.pdf. Accessed February 28, 2018.

Deficiency Needs Are Biological Needs

Applying the EBD model to Maslow's deficiency needs and the data from America's Promise Alliance suggests that unmet needs are potential precipitants of toxic stress. Given what we now know about the biological and developmental consequences of toxic stress responses to adversity, one might well argue that all of Maslow's deficiency needs are, in fact, biological needs and that the 5 promises provide a general outline of the essential biological needs of children.

Moreover, safe, stable, and nurturing relationships are the antidote to toxic stress because they meet the biological and safety needs of children (safe), they meet the love/connection needs of children (stable), and they meet the self-esteem needs of children (nurturing). In this way, safe, stable, and nurturing relationships meet the most basic biological needs of children, releasing the brake of toxic stress and providing children with the opportunity to self-actualize and to fulfill their endowed potential.

Box 6-2. Select Statistics for Unkept Promises (as of 2008 and Prior to the Affordable Care Act)

1. Have a healthy start.
   - More than one-third of teens and nearly one-fourth of younger children do not have health insurance coverage and annual visits to a doctor and a dentist—all critical components of good health care.
   - Although 80% to 90% of young people live in families with rules about eating healthy foods, nearly half still do not eat fruits and vegetables twice or more in a typical day.
2. Experience safe places.
   - One-fourth and one-third of all young people "never" or only "sometimes" feel safe at school and in their communities.
3. Have a caring adult.
   - One-third of teens and 20% of younger children do not have quality relationships with their parents.
   - More than 55% of adolescents and 40% of younger children do not have caring adults in all areas of their lives; that is, in their homes, schools, and communities.
4. Have opportunities to help others.
   - One-third of young people say they lack adult role models who volunteer and help others.
   - Forty percent of parents of children aged 6 to 17 years say they vote only some of the time.
   - Half of the parents of young people aged 6 to 17 years report that they rarely discuss current events with their children.
5. Have effective education.
   - More than 40% of parents of younger children and 66% of adolescents say their schools do not emphasize academic achievement.
   - Less than half of adolescents read for pleasure.
   - Almost 40% of adolescents do not have parents involved in their education.

There are many effective parenting techniques, but one could argue that providing safe, stable, and nurturing relationships to children is the fundamental basis for *good-enough* parenting.[19] Good-enough parenting is not saying that there is only one way to parent or that cultural or family values are unimportant. Good-enough parenting simply acknowledges that, regardless of other factors, children need safe, stable, and nurturing relationships to have a fair chance at self-actualization or the opportunity to fulfill their promise and potential. This concept will be discussed in more detail in the next chapter.

Beyond Good-Enough Parenting?

Meeting a child's deficiency needs is important because it releases an innate, intrinsic desire to self-actualize, but recall that self-actualization was not the ultimate goal for Maslow. He believed that some individuals are meta-motivated to move beyond self-actualization toward transcendence. With transcendence, individuals are able to find meaning and purpose beyond the confines of their own direct experience, in acts of altruism, the recognition of beauty, the pursuit of truth, or the awareness of their spiritual selves. Much as Maslow defined the deficiency needs of human life, Mark Bartel has defined the spiritual needs of human life.[20] Bartel, a well-respected clinical chaplain, argues that much of human psychological and spiritual suffering can be traced back to deficiencies in one or more of the following 5 areas: love, faith, hope, virtue, and beauty (Box 6-3).

Although there is some overlap between Bartel's spiritual needs and Maslow's deficiency needs, one way to reconcile these constructs is to reconsider the yin and yang of early childhood, protecting the brain and building new skills. In

Box 6-3. Bartel's Spiritual Needs

Love (Community, Connection)
- Affection, compassion
- Relationships, companionship
- Forgiveness, grace, mercy
- Self-worth, identity

Faith (Worldview)
- Personal philosophy
- Awe, wonder, humility
- Prayer, contact

Hope (Vision)
- Meaning, purpose
- Courage
- Perseverance

Virtue (Ethics)
- Integrity
- Character
- Goodness

Beauty (Renewal)
- Art, music
- Creativity
- Renewal
- Humor

general, meeting Maslow's deficiency needs protects the brain by minimizing significant adversity and potential precipitants of toxic stress, whereas fulfilling Bartel's spiritual needs builds the skills necessary for handling adversity in a healthy, adaptive manner (what is often termed *resilience*). For example, Bartel argues that fulfilling the spiritual need for love leads to compassion, mercy, and self-worth, which are critical attributes for responding to adversity in a healthy, restorative (rather than punitive or retributive) manner. Meeting the spiritual need for faith leads to prayer, introspection, and humility, all of which are important characteristics when dealing with significant adversity in a thoughtful, constructive way. Fulfilling the spiritual need for hope leads to purpose, courage, and perseverance, whereas fulfilling the spiritual need for virtue leads to integrity, character, and goodness. Meeting the spiritual need for beauty leads to art, music, and humor, which are potential passions, healthy distractions, and appropriate ways to cope with adversity. Regardless of one's religious background, the characteristics associated with the fulfillment of Bartel's spiritual needs are markers of resilience in that they all allow for appropriate, constructive, and healthy ways to respond to adversity.

Summary

The advances in developmental science presented in Part 1 reinforce century-old observations about the unfolding of development and the intrinsic drive to master. All of Maslow's deficiency needs (physiologic, safety, connection, self-esteem) are biological needs because, when they are not met, they precipitate a physiologic stress response that could become toxic. Policies and programs that fulfill the 5 promises of America's Promise Alliance and meet Maslow's deficiency needs or Bartel's spiritual needs are not just feel-good efforts. They are tangible steps toward the realization of children who are healthy; families that provide safe, stable, and nurturing relationships for their children; and communities that value and promote equal opportunity.

References

1. Richmond JB. Child development: a basic science for pediatrics. *Pediatrics.* 1967;39(5):649–658
2. Ross JB, McLaughlin MM. *The Portable Medieval Reader.* New York, NY: Viking Press; 1949
3. Halfon N, Inkelas M, Hochstein M. The health development organization: an organizational approach to achieving child health development. *Milbank Q.* 2000;78(3):447–497, 341
4. Tottenham N, Hare TA, Quinn BT, et al. Prolonged institutional rearing is associated with atypically large amygdala volume and difficulties in emotion regulation. *Dev Sci.* 2010;13(1):46–61
5. Lupien SJ, Parent S, Evans AC, et al. Larger amygdala but no change in hippocampal volume in 10-year-old children exposed to maternal depressive symptomatology since birth. *Proc Natl Acad Sci U S A.* 2011;108(34):14324–14329

6. Kim P, Evans GW, Angstadt M, et al. Effects of childhood poverty and chronic stress on emotion regulatory brain function in adulthood. *Proc Natl Acad Sci U S A.* 2013;110(46):18442–18447

7. Tottenham N, Hare TA, Millner A, Gilhooly T, Zevin JD, Casey BJ. Elevated amygdala response to faces following early deprivation. *Dev Sci.* 2011;14(2):190–204

8. VanTieghem MR, Tottenham N. Neurobiological programming of early life stress: functional development of amygdala-prefrontal circuitry and vulnerability for stress-related psychopathology. *Curr Top Behav Neurosci.* 2017

9. Silvers JA, Lumian DS, Gabard-Durnam L, et al. Previous institutionalization is followed by broader amygdala-hippocampal-PFC network connectivity during aversive learning in human development. *J Neurosci.* 2016;36(24):6420–6430

10. Shonkoff JP. Protecting brains, not simply stimulating minds. *Science.* 2011;333(6045):982–983

11. Montessori M. *The Absorbent Mind.* New York, NY: Henry Holt; 1995

12. Montessori M. *Childhood Education.* Chicago, IL: Regnery; 1974

13. Maria Montessori quotes. BrainyQuote Web site. https://www.brainyquote.com/quotes/maria_montessori_403453. Accessed February 28, 2018

14. Goldstein K. *The Organism, a Holistic Approach to Biology Derived From Pathological Data in Man.* New York, NY: American Book Co; 1939

15. Maslow AH. *Motivation and Personality.* New York, NY: Harper; 1954

16. Maslow AH. *The Farther Reaches of Human Nature.* New York, NY: Viking Press; 1971

17. Abraham Maslow quotes. BrainyQuote Web site. https://www.brainyquote.com/quotes/abraham_maslow_408724. Accessed February 28, 2018

18. America's Promise Alliance. *Every Child, Every Promise: Turning Failure Into Action.* Washington, DC: America's Promise Alliance; 2006. http://www.americaspromise.org/sites/default/files/d8/Every%20Child%20Every%20Promise%20-%20Full%20Report.pdf. Accessed February 28, 2018

19. Bettelheim B. *A Good Enough Parent: A Book on Child-rearing.* New York, NY: Knopf; 1987

20. Bartel M. What is spiritual? What is spiritual suffering? *J Pastoral Care Counsel.* 2004;58(3):187–201

Chapter 7

Supporting Parents and Caregivers

In order to develop normally, a child requires progressively more complex joint activity with one or more adults who have an irrational emotional relationship with the child. Somebody's got to be crazy about that kid. That's number one. First, last and always.

— Urie Bronfenbrenner (Cofounder of Head Start)[1]

The science underlying the ecobiodevelopmental (EBD) model explains how early childhood ecology is biologically embedded within the young child's genome and brain, and how that ecology influences behavior, learning, and health across the life span. Within that early childhood ecology, no factors are more pivotal than the young child's parents and caregivers. Although the focus of this chapter is on parents, this term is not intended to refer exclusively to a child's biological mother and father. Throughout this chapter, the term *parent* could also refer to foster parents, adoptive parents, grandparents, aunts, uncles, neighbors, and other adult caregivers who, in the words of Urie Bronfenbrenner, are "crazy about that kid."[1]

As discussed in the previous chapter, the advances in developmental science that support the EBD model also affirm a broader conception of the essential biological needs of children. Certainly, a child's physiologic needs, like clean water, nutritious food, and sufficient sleep, must be met for a child to self-actualize and fulfill his or her potential. But the neurobiology of toxic stress demonstrates that a child must also feel safe because fear activates the amygdala and inhibits the prefrontal cortex and hippocampus, making learning, the adoption of adaptive behaviors, and self-actualization more difficult.[2] The neurobiology of toxic stress demonstrates that a child must also feel loved, understood, and appreciated because safe, stable, and nurturing relationships shut down the amygdala, releasing its brake on the prefrontal cortex and hippocampus (see Figure 4-3).[3] Finally, we know that early brain and child development are reiterative processes that build on previous neuronal connections and behaviors to develop new neuronal pathways and skills.[4] Hence, a child must also feel nurtured, encouraged, and recognized for their efforts and progress, which not only supports the self-esteem needed to self-actualize but often softens the blow when the child's efforts or behaviors fall short. These are the essential biological needs of young children; when these deficiency needs are not met, it is simply much harder for children to self-actualize and fulfill their potential.

Given that all young children have these most basic biological needs, what does this mean for parents and caregivers of all varieties? Given that most, if not all, parents want their children to thrive, what are the barriers that prevent parents from meeting their children's most basic needs? Given that safe, stable, and nurturing relationships between 2 generations are needed to give young children a fair chance at fulfilling their potential, are ongoing efforts that focus only on one generation missing a fundamental element? This chapter will explore these important implications of the EBD model for parents and other caregivers.

Redefining the Concept of Good-Enough Parenting

The concept of *good-enough parenting* is not a new one,[5] and the phrase has been applied in many different ways.[6–9] For our purposes, we apply this moniker to the relationships and efforts required to meet a young child's most basic biological needs as discussed in the previous chapter (ie, physiologic, safety, connection, self-esteem). Having at least one good-enough parent is necessary for children to fulfill their potential. That said, good-enough parenting is insufficient to ensure a child's success because, ultimately, the emerging adolescent and eventual adult controls his or her own destiny. But being a good-enough parent allows that child to have a fair shot at self-actualization by ensuring that the child's needs are met in a developmentally appropriate manner.

Being good enough is not about *raising the ceiling* or defining a gold standard. Given the wide variation in cultural norms and values attached to parenting, there will be no universally acknowledged best parenting approach. But biology is universal, and good-enough parents strive to meet these most basic biological needs. Being good enough is about *raising the floor* and defining the bare minimum that all children need to have a fair shot at fulfilling their potential.

Being good enough recognizes that parents are only human and, therefore, are flawed from the start. There are no perfect parents and, despite our best efforts, there will be no perfect children. But by being good enough, parents and caregivers are building the safe, stable, and nurturing relationships that meet a young child's deficiency needs and release the brake on the child's intrinsic drive to develop, master, and succeed.

Parental Barriers to Relational Health

With more than a half-century of combined experience as pediatricians, we will testify that very few parents are determined to fail for their children. In our experience, almost all parents genuinely want their children to thrive and fulfill their potential. Yet, as discussed in the previous chapter, far too many children in the United States do not have their most basic needs or promises met. So why is there such a large disconnect between what we know and what we do?

For better or for worse, intentionally or subconsciously, parents tend to raise their children the way their parents raised them.[10] As adults, we are inclined to do what we know, and what we know is what we have observed, experienced, or learned in the past. But our past is not our destiny! One of the principal objectives of this book is to educate not only practicing physicians but parents, caregivers, educators, policy makers, and legislators about the advances in developmental science, the EBD model, and the way that early childhood experiences affect life course trajectories. The EBD model suggests that it all comes down to *relational health:* when good-enough parents develop safe, stable, and nurturing relationships with their children, they are laying the foundation for lifelong health. Given this understanding, we are well positioned not only to prevent suboptimal outcomes but to actually build brains, strengthen families, and create communities that care for each other.

But how, in a tangible way, do communities, health care professionals, and parents collectively promote the safe, stable, and nurturing relationships that meet a young child's most basic biological needs and release the brake on the child's innate drive to develop, master, and self-actualize? All parents, to one degree or another, face daily barriers to developing safe, stable, and nurturing relationships with their children. Most parents are confronted with limitations on their time, material resources, and/or energy, and these limitations all too often constrain their most sincere intentions to be the best possible versions of themselves for their children. Fortunately, most kids are resilient. If their deficiency needs are met, and if they have the benefit of at least one safe, stable, and nurturing relationship, most children will thrive.[3,11]

Parental Adverse Childhood Experiences

But to be fair, some parents face more limitations than others. All parents were once children themselves, and those who experienced high levels of childhood adversity and toxic stress may have a larger and more active amygdala, making them more prone to impulsivity, emotionality, and aggression. They may have long forgotten their adversity as a child, but implicit memories can be triggered by their young child's experiences, resulting in overwhelming and confusing emotional responses to seemingly innocuous everyday events. Recall that the amygdala also inhibits the activity of the prefrontal cortex, making executive functions, like emotional regulation, impulse inhibition, abstract thought, and planning, harder to accomplish. Clearly, these tendencies have the potential to affect an adult's parenting style, as well as their ability to form safe, stable, and nurturing relationships with not only their children but their spouses, neighbors, and coworkers. This is *not* saying that all adults who experienced childhood adversity or toxic stress are destined to have difficulty with parenting and relational health. But it is an acknowledgment that early childhood adversity and toxic stress have the potential to negatively affect parenting skills and relational supports. Briefly stated, it is simply harder, but certainly not impossible, for parents to develop safe, stable, and nurturing relationships with their children if they never experienced safe, stable, and nurturing relationships themselves.

Parental Deficiency Needs

As discussed in Part 1, adults who experienced early childhood adversity and toxic stress are at higher risk of having poor physical and mental health, fractured social networks (eg, divorce), and job insecurity.[12,13] Consequently, parents who experienced significant adversity as a child might be faced with a one-two punch: they may have neurobiological and emotional baggage from their past (as discussed in the previous section), and they may currently be in survival mode because their essential needs (ie, physiology, safety, connectional, self-esteem) are not being met. If "being the best parent I can possibly be" is a measure of self-actualization, then Maslow and the biology of toxic stress would predict that realizing that potential is simply more onerous when the parent's biological needs are not met. Hence, parental food or housing insecurity, inadequate sleep, and chronic disease are potential barriers to parents developing safe, stable, and nurturing relationships with their children. Similarly, when parental safety needs are not met due to domestic or neighborhood violence; when parental connectional needs are not met due to divorce, limited access to extended family, or frequent moves; or when parental self-esteem needs are not met due to academic failure, unemployment, or poverty, they are potential barriers to relational health. Again, this is *not* saying that unmet parental needs make it impossible to be a good-enough parent. But it is an acknowledgment that when parents are in survival mode—when their deficiency needs are not being met—it is hard for parents to be in relational mode and to form the safe, stable, and nurturing relationships their children need at a basic biological level (Figure 7-1).

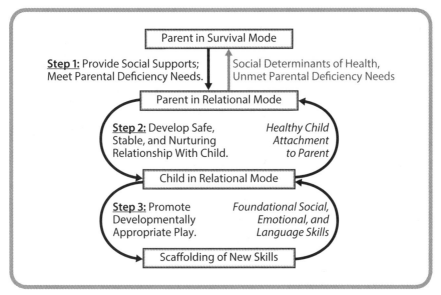

Figure 7-1. Helping parents to help their children includes at least 3 distinct steps. When parents are in survival mode, it is hard for them to form the safe, stable, and nurturing relationships (SSNRs) that protect the child's brain (releasing the brake) and promote the formation of new skills (stepping on the gas). Consequently, Step 1 is to move parents from survival mode into relational mode by meeting their deficiency needs and providing social supports. Conversely, unmet parental deficiency needs and the social determinants of health (gray arrow) are likely to shift parents back into survival mode. Once parents are in relational mode, Step 2 is to assist them in being engaged and responsive to their child to form the SSNRs that move the child into relational mode. Doing so minimizes toxic stress responses and promotes a healthy child attachment that, in turn, encourages the parent to remain in relational mode. Step 3 is to assist parents in playing with the child in a developmentally appropriate manner to note and encourage the child's new skills as they emerge. An early focus on foundational social, emotional, and language skills will allow the child to remain in relational mode. Note that once a parent is in relational mode, the fostering of a safe, stable, and nurturing relationship with the child; playing with the child in a developmentally appropriate manner; the child's emerging social, emotional, and language skills; and healthy child attachment with the parent all form a positively reinforcing cycle that encourages both the parent and the child to remain in relational mode. But the social determinants of health and unmet parental deficiency needs (gray arrow) threaten to derail this positively reinforcing cycle by shifting the parent back into survival mode.

Parental Challenges at Multiple Levels

Stated simply, parents who are struggling to fulfill their own needs often cannot adequately attend to the needs of their children. Parental struggles are protean, and parental challenges can be further categorized as personal, interpersonal, or societal (Box 7-1).

Unmet *personal* needs with the potential to impair the parent-child relationship include food insecurity, housing insecurity, job insecurity, and health insecurity. Personal challenges include maladaptive coping mechanisms and risky behaviors like substance abuse, alcohol abuse, and promiscuity. Struggling to meet these needs and overcome these challenges makes it more difficult, but certainly not impossible, for parents to be good enough and to meet their child's need for at least one safe, stable, and nurturing relationship.

Interpersonal challenges with the potential to impair a parent's ability to form safe, stable, and nurturing relationships with their children include divorce or single parenting, domestic violence, lack of support from extended family, and frequent moves that prevent friendly relations with neighbors. Social isolation is a potent inducer of toxic stress responses and poor overall health for children and adults.[14–17]

Box 7-1. Challenging Situations That May Affect the Ability of Parents to Form Safe, Stable, and Nurturing Relationships With Their Children

Personal
- Food insecurity
- Housing insecurity
- Job insecurity (inadequate employment or lack of employment)
- Health insecurity (active or chronic disease; inadequate health insurance)
- Risky behaviors (drug use, alcohol abuse, promiscuity; may be behavioral attempts to cope due to parental adversity as child)

Interpersonal
- Divorce or single parenting
- Domestic partner violence (acute, chronic, or remote)
- Lack of extended family
- Frequent moves and few social supports

Societal
- Educational disparities
- Economic inequities
- Neighborhood violence
- Racism/discrimination

Societal challenges with the potential to impair relational health include a wide range of risk factors that are collectively referred to as the *social determinants of health*. These include educational disparities, economic inequities, neighborhood violence, systemic discrimination, and racism.[18] These societal challenges also lead to social isolation, more toxic stress, and less adaptive functioning.

All too often, challenges at the personal, interpersonal, and societal levels are inextricably intertwined. Parents who are challenged in many ways at multiple levels are at higher risk for their own safety and well-being, and these families may need access to additional social, financial, and medical resources to meet their children's most basic needs. Doing so will not only assist the parents but improve the parents' ability to form the safe, stable, and nurturing relationships that their children need to become happy, healthy, and productive citizens, not to mention good-enough parents themselves someday. This is why the most successful interventions will be 2-generational.[19]

Two-Generational Approaches to Address the Effect of Poverty

Reframing sources of parental adversity as barriers to relational health reveals why 2-generational approaches are a necessity. For example, poverty makes it harder, but certainly not impossible, for parents to invest the time, energy, and resources into developing the safe, stable, and nurturing relationships that young children need to thrive at a basic biological level. Parents of low-income families speak, read, and play (singing or telling stories) with their children less frequently than parents in higher-income families.[20–22] As discussed in Chapter 4, the seminal work of Hart and Risley demonstrated that by the time they reach their fourth birthday, children in low-income families are exposed to 30 million fewer words than their peers in high-income families. In addition, they found that when young children in low-income families were engaged by their parents, the interactions tended to be more controlling and intrusive. More recent work by Shah and colleagues demonstrated that parents with the lowest incomes versus the highest incomes reported less frequent participation in activities like reading, singing, telling a story, or taking their child on an outing.[22] More importantly, less frequent participation in these activities was associated with an increased risk of delays in development. By no means does poverty make it impossible for parents to focus on relational health and the activities that foster safe, stable, and nurturing relationships—but it clearly makes it harder.

The good news is that 2-generational interventions that focus on relational health and fostering safe, stable, and nurturing relationships benefit child development—particularly for children in low-income families.[3,19] Although the Reach Out and Read program is known as an important intervention to promote early literacy, it also promotes the routine, developmentally appropriate interactions between parent and child that nurture new skills as they emerge.[23] Similarly, a longitudinal study on Jamaican children whose growth was retarded demonstrated that 2 years of weekly play sessions to improve the mother-child interactions during the first few years of life resulted in fewer fights, less violent behavior, higher IQ and educational attainment, and fewer symptoms of depression and social isolation when those children became adults.[24] Even modest increases to family income decrease childhood stress[25] and improve developmental outcomes,[26] presumably by decreasing parental stress and allowing for more parent-child interactions.[27,28] In fact, one could argue that, among the varied but few longitudinal interventions known to improve developmental outcomes (examples include the Nurse-Family Partnership,[29–32] the Perry preschool study,[33] the Abecedarian Project,[34] the Chicago Longitudinal Study,[35] and the Jamaican play study[24]), the one commonality is that they all included parental involvement in the child's development and early education.

Two Generations, But Many Opportunities

Parents are the primary influencers in the early life of a child. When parents encounter adversity, both generations may suffer if that adversity impairs the parents' ability to develop or maintain a safe, stable, and nurturing relationship with their child. The science underlying the EBD model helps us to define what the basic biological needs of young children are, as well as the essential elements of what makes parenting good enough. When the well-established barriers to good-enough parenting (ie, past parental adverse childhood experiences, current unmet needs, and parental challenges at the personal, interpersonal, and societal levels) are recognized as impediments to relational health, the need for 2-generational approaches becomes obvious.[3,19] As pediatricians, teachers, home visitors, community health workers, and other professionals who interact with young families, we must learn how to help the parents to help their children (see Figure 7-1). Family-centered pediatric medical homes cannot accomplish this lofty objective in a vacuum. Improving early childhood ecology and life course outcomes for generations to come will require collaborative, working relationships between the medical home and community resources like parent support groups, income and employment assistance, shelters, food pantries, legal aid, and early education and child care centers. Consequently, the next chapter will consider the implications of the EBD model for communities as a whole.

References

1. National Scientific Council on the Developing Child. *Young Children Develop in an Environment of Relationships: Working Paper No. 1.* 2004. http://developingchild.harvard.edu/resources/wp1. Accessed February 28, 2018

2. National Scientific Council on the Developing Child. *Persistent Fear and Anxiety Can Affect Young Children's Learning and Development: Working Paper No. 9.* 2010. https://developingchild.harvard.edu/resources/persistent-fear-and-anxiety-can-affect-young-childrens-learning-and-development. Accessed February 28, 2018

3. Center on the Developing Child at Harvard University. *Supportive Relationships and Active Skill-Building Strengthen the Foundations of Resilience: Working Paper No. 13.* 2015. https://developingchild.harvard.edu/resources/supportive-relationships-and-active-skill-building-strengthen-the-foundations-of-resilience. Accessed February 28, 2018

4. National Scientific Council on the Developing Child. *The Timing and Quality of Early Experiences Combine to Shape Brain Architecture: Working Paper No. 5.* 2007. https://developingchild.harvard.edu/resources/the-timing-and-quality-of-early-experiences-combine-to-shape-brain-architecture. Accessed February 28, 2018

5. Winnicott DW. *The Child, the Family, and the Outside World.* 2nd ed. New York, NY: Perseus Publishing; 1992

6. Bettelheim B. *A Good Enough Parent: A Book on Child-rearing.* New York, NY: Knopf; 1987

7. Louis JP, Louis KM. *Good Enough Parenting: An In-Depth Perspective on Meeting Core Emotional Needs and Avoiding Exasperation.* Garden City, NY: Morgan James Publishing; 2015

8. Hoghughi M, Speight AN. Good enough parenting for all children—a strategy for a healthier society. *Arch Dis Child.* 1998;78(4):293–296

9. Gilsdorf JR. The good-enough parent. *JAMA.* 2016;316(20):2089

10. Lomanowska AM, Boivin M, Hertzman C, Fleming AS. Parenting begets parenting: a neurobiological perspective on early adversity and the transmission of parenting styles across generations. *Neuroscience.* 2017;342:120–139

11. America's Promise Alliance. *Every Child, Every Promise: Turning Failure Into Action.* Washington, DC: America's Promise Alliance; 2006. http://www.americaspromise.org/sites/default/files/d8/Every%20Child%20Every%20Promise%20-%20Full%20Report.pdf. Accessed February 28, 2018

12. Anda RF, Felitti VJ, Bremner JD, et al. The enduring effects of abuse and related adverse experiences in childhood. A convergence of evidence from neurobiology and epidemiology. *Eur Arch Psychiatry Clin Neurosci.* 2006;256(3):174–186

13. Felitti VJ, Anda RF, Nordenberg D, et al. Relationship of childhood abuse and household dysfunction to many of the leading causes of death in adults. The Adverse Childhood Experiences (ACE) Study. *Am J Prev Med.* 1998;14(4):245–258

14. Pantell M, Rehkopf D, Jutte D, Syme SL, Balmes J, Adler N. Social isolation: a predictor of mortality comparable to traditional clinical risk factors. *Am J Public Health.* 2013;103(11):2056–2062

15. Koss KJ, Hostinar CE, Donzella B, Gunnar MR. Social deprivation and the HPA axis in early development. *Psychoneuroendocrinology.* 2014;50:1–13

16. Fries AB, Shirtcliff EA, Pollak SD. Neuroendocrine dysregulation following early social deprivation in children. *Dev Psychobiol.* 2008;50(6):588–599

17. Grant N, Hamer M, Steptoe A. Social isolation and stress-related cardiovascular, lipid, and cortisol responses. *Ann Behav Med.* 2009;37(1):29–37

18. Berger M, Sarnyai Z. "More than skin deep": stress neurobiology and mental health consequences of racial discrimination. *Stress.* 2015;18(1):1–10

19. Zuckerman B. Two-generation pediatric care: a modest proposal. *Pediatrics.* 2016;137(1):1–5

20. Hart B, Risley TR. *The Social World of Children Learning to Talk.* Baltimore, MD: Paul H. Brookes Publishing Co; 1999

21. Hart B, Risley TR. *Meaningful Differences in the Everyday Experience of Young American Children.* Baltimore, MD: Paul H. Brookes Publishing Co; 1995

22. Shah R, Sobotka SA, Chen YF, Msall ME. Positive parenting practices, health disparities, and developmental progress. *Pediatrics.* 2015;136(2):318–326

23. Zuckerman B, Khandekar A. Reach Out and Read: evidence based approach to promoting early child development. *Curr Opin Pediatr.* 2010;22(4):539–544

24. Walker SP, Chang SM, Vera-Hernández M, Grantham-McGregor S. Early childhood stimulation benefits adult competence and reduces violent behavior. *Pediatrics.* 2011;127(5):849–857

25. Fernald LC, Gunnar MR. Poverty-alleviation program participation and salivary cortisol in very low-income children. *Soc Sci Med.* 2009;68(12):2180–2189

26. Ozer EJ, Fernald LC, Manley JG, Gertler PJ. Effects of a conditional cash transfer program on children's behavior problems. *Pediatrics.* 2009;123(4):e630–e637

27. Sherr L, Macedo A, Tomlinson M, Skeen S, Cluver LD. Could cash and good parenting affect child cognitive development? A cross-sectional study in South Africa and Malawi. *BMC Pediatr.* 2017;17(1):123

28. Cash transfers for children—investing into the future. *Lancet.* 2009;373(9682):2172

29. Eckenrode J, Campa M, Luckey DW, et al. Long-term effects of prenatal and infancy nurse home visitation on the life course of youths: 19-year follow-up of a randomized trial. *Arch Pediatr Adolesc Med.* 2010;164(1):9–15

30. Kitzman HJ, Olds DL, Cole RE, et al. Enduring effects of prenatal and infancy home visiting by nurses on children: follow-up of a randomized trial among children at age 12 years. *Arch Pediatr Adolesc Med.* 2010;164(5):412–418

31. Donelan-McCall N, Eckenrode J, Olds DL. Home visiting for the prevention of child maltreatment: lessons learned during the past 20 years. *Pediatr Clin North Am.* 2009;56(2):389–403

32. Zielinski DS, Eckenrode J, Olds DL. Nurse home visitation and the prevention of child maltreatment: impact on the timing of official reports. *Dev Psychopathol.* 2009;21(2):441–453

33. Schweinhart LJ, Montie J, Xiang Z, Barnett WS, Belfield CR, Nores M. *Lifetime Effects: The High/Scope Perry Preschool Study Through Age 40.* Ypsilanti, MI: High/Scope Press; 2005

34. Campbell F, Conti G, Heckman JJ, et al. Early childhood investments substantially boost adult health. *Science.* 2014;343(6178):1478–1485

35. Reynolds AJ, Temple JA, Ou SR, Arteaga IA, White BA. School-based early childhood education and age-28 well-being: effects by timing, dosage, and subgroups. *Science.* 2011;333(6040):360–364

Chapter 8

The Role of Communities

According to the ecobiodevelopmental (EBD) model, the ongoing but cumulative dance between nurture (ecology) and nature (genome) drives development, not only in childhood but across the life span. To improve life-course trajectories, the most productive efforts will go toward improving the early childhood ecology. In Chapter 6, we discussed how a child's unmet needs (ie, physiologic, safety, connection, and esteem) can precipitate a toxic stress response, placing a brake on the child's innate drive to self-actualize. Meeting a child's essential needs through the provision of a safe, stable, and nurturing relationship releases a brake on development, allowing children to fulfill their potential.

Fortunately, most parents are able to provide their children with safe, stable, and nurturing relationships and to meet their children's most essential needs. But in Chapter 7, we discussed that some parents have their own unmet needs and it may be difficult for parents who never benefitted from safe, stable, and nurturing relationships in their own childhood to develop those relationships with their children. In essence, it is hard to give something you never received. Two-generational approaches that address the parents' and child's needs are, therefore, necessary to improve the younger generation's medical, educational, and economic outcomes.

This chapter will focus on the role the larger community plays in helping parents to help their children. As in previous chapters, we will apply a public health framework that recognizes there will be no single magic bullet intervention, but that layered or nested interventions can have a collective effect on parents and their children. Such a framework also acknowledges that not all families are in need of the same level of support, but all families benefit from community supports to one degree or another. Just as families are well positioned to nurture wellness in their children, local communities have ample opportunities to nurture wellness in their families.

Opportunities at the Community Level

A public health approach that addresses childhood toxic stress and promotes childhood wellness at the community level acknowledges at least 3 different types of opportunity (Figure 8-1). At the top of the public health pyramid, there are opportunities for communities to *meet the unmet needs of parents and their children.* In the middle, there are opportunities for communities to *identify and support those parents and children at risk* for significant adversity or unmet needs. Finally, at the base of the pyramid, there are opportunities for communities to *support relational health and wellness in a proactive, universal manner.*

Two-Generational Approach to Unmet Needs

Unmet needs have a negative effect on a child's biology and a parent's functioning, but communities frequently have the collective resources needed to assist families in meeting these most basic needs. For example, communities have used food pantries and homeless shelters to address unmet physiologic needs like food insecurity and a quiet place to sleep. They have addressed unmet safety needs, like bullying and intimate partner violence, through school-based programs,[1,2] public awareness campaigns,[3,4] and the training of police on how to

Public Health Level	Types of Prevention	Community Approaches	Examples
3	Tertiary	Meet unmet deficiency needs of parents and children.	Food pantries, crisis shelters, free medical clinics
2	Secondary	Identify and support parents and children at risk for adversity.	Home visiting, parenting support, early intervention
1	Primary	Support relational health and wellness in a universal manner.	Universal preschool, parks, playgrounds, recreation leagues

Figure 8-1. Applying a public health framework to community approaches that will promote childhood and family wellness.

assess lethality and how to confidentially connect those at risk with safe houses and legal supports.[5] For youth who are isolated, alienated, or disenfranchised, some communities have invested in peer-led support groups, specialized summer camps, and mentoring programs like Big Brothers Big Sisters of America to encourage more connectedness. To promote adult connectedness, some communities have embraced welcome committees for immigrants, reentry programs to support the integration of offenders recently released from incarceration, adult recreational leagues in neighborhoods with violence,[6,7] home visiting programs for first-time mothers,[8,9] and Centering Pregnancy programs for impoverished mothers-to-be.[10,11] To address unmet needs for youth self-esteem, communities have intentionally developed opportunities for youth to contribute,[12,13] whereas adult self-esteem might be addressed through job training and volunteer programs.[14–19] When these essential needs (ie, physiologic, safety, connection, and self-esteem) are not met, fewer parents and their children will fulfill their biological, educational, and economic potential. Opportunities to address 2-generational needs should be viewed as essential for communities interested in raising their academic standing, decreasing gaps in their social services, and improving their measures of population-level health (eg, the prevalence of obesity or depression).

Identifying and Supporting Those Families Most at Risk

Communities have multiple points of contact with families because young families often make use of services from the health care, education, civil service, and business sectors (Figure 8-2). Each of these sectors is well placed

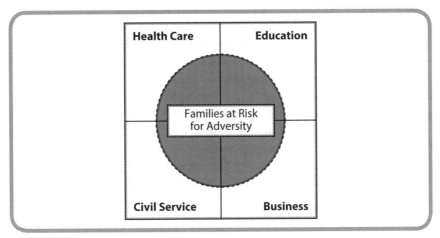

Figure 8-2. Because many community sectors (including the health care, education, civil service, and business sectors) have points of contact with families at risk for adversity, they provide opportunities for identification and support.

to identify families who might be at risk for adversity due to any number of concerns. For example, the health care community might be aware of a serious illness or death in the family. The education sector might be alarmed to notice that the children in one particular family are absent frequently or not performing up to grade level. The civil service sector might be concerned because neighbors have been reporting loud arguments or suspected animal abuse in the home. And the business community might be concerned because of recent layoffs at the neighborhood factory. Given concerns about confidentiality, it may not be feasible for all these sectors to coordinate their care for the benefit of the family or child unless written consent is obtained. But any of these sectors could easily refer a family to community service agencies that provide case management and link families at risk with locally available supports.[20] The United Way frequently supports these community service agencies,[21] and local communities interested in addressing early childhood adversity and toxic stress will recognize the important role these organizations play in preventing and addressing unmet needs.

Supporting Relational Health in a Proactive, Universal Manner

Local communities and their leaders deal with a wide array of constituencies, as discussed previously, including the health care, education, business, and social (civil) service sectors. The ability of communities and their leaders to interact in positive ways for the betterment of all requires—no surprise here— relational health! As the adage says, "If you want to go far, go together." But going together requires, at the very least, 1) a shared or common vision that is embraced by a variety of constituencies that are all too frequently at odds with each other; 2) the synergy that occurs when a wide array of constituencies work collaboratively to achieve unanimous measures of success; and 3) clear, consistent messaging to remind the constituencies, policy makers, and public what the vision and measures of success are.

One of the primary objectives of this book is to detail what that shared vision of community life could be, if it were to be grounded in the latest advances in developmental science. A development-informed vision would recognize not only the long-term and intergenerational transfer of toxic stress but the potential for early safe, stable, and nurturing relationships to positively influence health outcomes, educational success, and economic productivity for decades to come. As mentioned in Chapter 1, there is only one science of early brain and child development, but it has implications for the health, educational success, and prosperity of our communities for decades to come.

A development-informed vision recognizes that to improve a multitude of outcomes across the life span, efforts must be made to improve the early childhood ecology. It acknowledges that to mitigate the biology (eg, epigenetics, neuroscience, behavioral allostasis) underlying well-established disparities in health, education, and wealth, potential deficiency needs must be addressed in a 2-generational manner. As Nicholas Kristof has written, "Talent is universal, but opportunity is not."[22,23] A development-informed vision does not ignore disparities in opportunity or inequities in the provision of deficiency needs; nor does it degenerate into fruitless finger-pointing about who is responsible (eg, child, parents, neighborhood, government, society as a whole). It does not advocate for the "redistribution of wealth" but, rather, for the "pre-distribution of wealth"[24] by making significant investments in families with young children to ensure that their essential needs are met and the early childhood ecology promotes the formation of safe, stable, and nurturing relationships.

But to bring this shared vision to fruition will require a collective, collaborative approach that extends across sectors and constituencies. All too often, distinct groups within communities champion their own most pressing concerns without acknowledging the way that their concerns are linked inextricably to the concerns of the other constituencies, or the way that a collective, collaborative approach might improve the relational health of the entire community. For example, the business community might have legitimate concerns about a lack of well-educated, healthy, and productive employees, but the health care sector is concerned primarily about opioid abuse or obesity. At the same time, the local social service agencies are focused on battling the effects of unemployment and poverty, while the schools are concerned about falling test scores and rising dropout rates. The EBD framework helps these distinct constituencies understand how their concerns are intrinsically related to the concerns of the other sectors. To achieve the broad developmental outcomes embraced by a wide array of constituencies (ie, happy, healthy, well-educated, and productive citizens), the EBD framework suggests that communities work collaboratively to improve the early childhood ecology by collectively committing to meet deficiency needs and promote relational health in a universal manner.

Finally, building a shared vision and implementing a collective approach to fulfill that vision requires clear, consistent messaging about community norms for acceptable behaviors and outcomes. Messaging that is precise and unwavering allows for trust to develop, empathy to be shared, and common goals and measures to be sought. A good example of the power of consistent messaging is found in the work of the Communities That Care (CTC) project.[25–29] The CTC project is an evidence-based approach endorsed by the US Substance Abuse and Mental Health Services Administration to address a wide array of adolescent problem behaviors, including substance abuse, violence, truancy, and teen pregnancy. The CTC project is based on social development theory and research that demonstrates the 5 basic factors needed to promote positive social development.

1. Developmentally appropriate opportunities for youth involvement in the community's betterment efforts
2. Promoting youth skill formation
3. Community recognition for youth efforts, improvement, and achievement
4. Strong social bonds between youth and adults
5. Clear, consistent messaging from all community stakeholders to set the social norms for specific behaviors

Returning to Maslow's deficiency needs, factor 4 addresses the biological need for connectedness, and factors 1, 2, and 3 address the biological need for esteem. What the CTC project adds is factor 5—the clear, consistent messaging for the community's standards of behavior.

The CTC project suggests that for positive developmental outcomes, communities must carefully consider how they convey their standards about the provision of biologically requisite needs and the importance of relational health. Are clean water, nutritious food, and adequate sleep simply commodities available to those who can afford them, or is inequity in their provision an unacceptable breach of relational health? For safety, is violence narrowly defined in terms of physical harm, or does violence in all its varied forms (eg, physical, emotional, racial, gender based, economic) reflect a fundamental breakdown in relational health? For connectedness, should parents use corporal punishment, or should they be encouraged to embrace parenting techniques that maintain a positive parent-child relationship?[30,31] Similarly, should local judges rely solely on punitive or retributive measures, or should they be encouraged to embrace the principles of restorative justice?[32–35] For esteem, should opportunities to participate in the arts, music, and sports be available only to those who can afford to pay to play, or should schools acknowledge the need for all youth to contribute and excel in one medium or another?

The CTC project also highlights the importance of promoting youth skill formation (basic factor 2). Ross Greene, noted psychologist and author of several books,[36,37] including *Raising Human Beings,*[38] argues that youth who can do well, will do well. But when youth are struggling, there is usually a disconnect between our expectations and the child's actual skill level. Greene argues that additional motivators, like sticker charts and punishments, are not likely to succeed if the child is simply deficient in one requisite skill or another. He argues that it is only through connectedness and safe, stable, and nurturing relationships that adults are able to decipher which rudimentary skills are lacking. That connectedness also becomes the trusted foundation that encourages the youth to build deficient skills through family-based, classroom-based, extracurricular, or community-based opportunities. In many instances, it is not solely cognitive skills that are missing but the social-emotional, language, and adaptive skills necessary for relational health. Ultimately, the building of community wellness requires consistent messaging regarding the foundational importance of relational health.

Moving Communities Forward: Change Begins With Me

Health care futurist Leland Kaiser has been quoted as stating that for anything happening in a community, citizens should acknowledge that "I am the problem; I am the solution; I am the resource."[39] These simple 12 words force us to acknowledge our individual culpability when children fail to achieve their potential. But they also empower us to work collaboratively to promote relational health and wellness. This challenge serves as a useful call to action, as well as the starting point for moving communities forward.

Citizenship demands that we actively engage in opportunities to improve our communities, and advocating for children and their families is one powerful way to do so. When considering the components of such civic engagement at the individual level, a specific paradigm has been previously suggested.[39] The 5 steps toward community improvement are

1. Be the best parent you can be.
2. Get involved in community activities that promote relational health.
3. Stay involved.
4. Love others.
5. Forgive others.

These 5 steps reflect the interactional, relational nature of civic engagement. Parenting in modern society is often based on the parent's childhood experiences and augmented by the norms found within the parent's current peer group. The many facets of contemporary parenting are protean (eg, what constitutes healthy nutrition, when are daily routines too busy, what is developmentally appropriate play, how can discipline always be positive, how can cyberbullying be prevented), and parents frequently wonder if what they are doing is the best way or if they are messing up their children. Disseminating consistent messages about the notion of good-enough parenting, providing for essential needs, and communicating the foundational importance of relational health will require citizens who are involved, loving, and full of forgiveness—even if others might question their intentions, political leanings, or value systems.

Civic engagement is a 2-fold process. First, one needs to recognize the wide array of community activities that might promote relational health, identify which of these activities matches well with one's passions and skill set, and get involved by volunteering or advocating. The second, often more difficult, step is to sustain this involvement when there are interpersonal conflicts, fundamental differences in vision for the activity, or major setbacks, like the end of a program's pilot funding. Staying involved implies a willingness to adapt to change, to be a part of the process, and to think creatively.

A love for others might well be considered the foundation for all civic engagement, but all too often, righteous indignation, intolerance, and poor conflict resolution creep into our interactions and erode our collective relational health. Without the recognition of these failings and an acknowledgment that "I am the problem," we cannot move forward to enhance the lives of our fellow citizens.

Although the concept of forgiveness may not be synonymous with civic engagement, the practice of forgiveness is a critical step toward community improvement. Forgiveness is a developmental process because asking for and extending forgiveness is different at almost every age.[40–42] But at any age, forgiveness is grounded in the ability to accept our common fallibility and humanity. Vulnerability, sincerity, humility, reconciliation, and an openness to change are the qualities that make the practice of forgiveness so difficult, yet so vital, for relational health and civic engagement. These qualities are also necessary for the practice of communal forgiveness. Groups or organizations must be able to acknowledge their breaches in relational health, even if they were perpetrated in the past by different people.[43,44] With such acknowledgments, communities are able to restore relational health and move forward collaboratively.

These 5 steps (ie, be a good-enough parent, get involved, stay involved, love others, and forgive others) represent a potential path for individuals to become more engaged in their community's efforts to help parents help their children.

Moving Communities Forward: Collective Efforts to Address Unequal Opportunity

Assuming that a community has an engaged citizenry that shares a development-informed vision for the betterment of their community, how does the community begin to move forward collaboratively?

In his book *Our Kids: The American Dream in Crisis,*[45] Robert D. Putnam argues that inequity is the place to start. Putnam identifies and delineates a disturbing opportunity gap for numerous children and families. Children from less-advantaged neighborhoods are more likely to have family disruption (eg, younger parents, single parents, lower employment rates, higher rates of incarceration), parenting difficulties (eg, educational inequalities, greater stress, fewer child development opportunities), schooling disparities (eg, fewer academic and athletic opportunities, gaps in educational achievement), and depleted community resources (eg, diminished social networks, fewer mentors, less neighborhood trust, decreased church attendance) than their peers in more privileged communities. Putnam argues that this opportunity gap threatens upward mobility and challenges the American dream that every child has a fair shot at a bright future. Similarly, we have argued that unmet deficiency needs make the very concept of "equal opportunity" a biological fallacy.

Restoring the American dream and fulfilling the promise of equal opportunity hinges on a fundamental shift in the way communities view their most treasured resource: their children. Are all children in the community "our kids"? Or are "my kids" distinct from "those kids"? Is there a shared responsibility for the welfare of all the children in the community? If so, unmet needs and opportunity gaps are simply untenable, and their very existence is a threat to the relational health of the entire community. Collaborative, 2-generational efforts are needed to provide for unmet needs, close opportunity gaps, and improve the life course trajectories of the next generation.

Building on his previous work (*Bowling Alone: The Collapse and Revival of American Community*),[46] Putnam suggests many community improvements to address unequal opportunity. He categorizes them under the headings of *family structure, child development and parenting, schools,* and *community* (Box 8-1). Examples of community-based efforts to improve *family structure* could include enhancing access to counseling before marriage, increasing the availability of contraception, and increasing economic incentives for employment and child support. To support *child development and parenting,* communities could increase access to quality preschools, support robust home visiting programs, and enhance access to peer-led parent support groups and parent trainers. Community-based opportunities to address inequities through *schools* include minimizing residential segregation and promoting neighborhood inclusion; reducing suspensions and expulsions by using restorative, rather than punitive measures; and promoting and enhancing opportunities at local community colleges. Finally, inequities could be addressed at the *community* level through programs that encourage a communal sense of responsibility for each other, promote the use of mentoring, support inclusive faith communities, and invest in neglected neighborhoods. For communities with a development-informed vision and a desire to tackle inequities in opportunity, the list in Box 8-1 could serve as a potential blueprint for moving forward, with the acknowledged caveat

Box 8-1. Suggested Community Improvements to Address Unequal Opportunity

Family Structure
- Enhance access to counseling before marriage and increase the availability of contraception.
- Increase economic incentives for employment and child support.
- Advocate for federal and state tax policies that increase after-tax family income (eg, expand the earned income tax credit and the child tax credit).
- Protect child poverty programs (eg, school lunches, Children's Health Insurance Program).
- Reduce incarceration for nonviolent crimes and enhance rehabilitation.

Child Development and Parenting
- Increase access to quality child care (0–3 years old).
- Encourage preschool programs (3 years old–kindergarten).
- Support robust home visiting programs.
- Promote early reading programs (eg, Reach Out and Read).
- Enhance access to parent support groups and parent trainers.

Schools
- Minimize residential segregation and promote inclusion.
- Encourage parental engagement in schools.
- Engage community resources/businesses as partners with schools.
- Reduce suspensions and expulsions (restorative over punitive measures).
- Promote and enhance opportunities at community colleges.

Community
- Encourage a communal sense of responsibility for each other.
- Increase and share the local social capital.
- Promote mentoring programs.
- Support inclusive faith communities.
- Invest in neglected neighborhoods, minimizing disparities.

Derived from Putnam RD. *Our Kids: The American Dream in Crisis.* New York, NY: Simon & Schuster; 2015.

that each community has its own unique strengths, untapped resources, and areas most in need of improvement. Figure 8-1 also provides some tangible examples of community-based efforts toward minimizing inequities and promoting childhood wellness.

Inequity Harms the Entire Community

Intriguingly, the negative effects of economic inequities are not limited to those individuals who have actually experienced poverty. According to data from the Organisation for Economic Co-operation and Development, the

World Bank, and others, the wider the degree of economic disparity experienced by a society (as measured by the Gini coefficient), the worse everyone in that society fares—including the wealthy.[47–50] This suggests that it is not just the lack of material goods that is harmful to a society's health; economic inequities may undermine the social connectedness and relational health that are needed for all to thrive.[51]

Empowerment

The EBD model, life course science, epigenetics, and developmental neuroscience reinforce sociological arguments for the need to engage communities to improve a wide array of outcomes. The development of children and the building of parenting skills are never accomplished in a void. Communities rise or fall on their ability to provide for their most vulnerable citizens: their children. Much like individuals who feel threatened, communities in survival mode are more likely to go alone and are less likely to embrace relational health. But development-informed communities will constantly look for ways to improve the lives of their children and families. It really does take a village to raise a child, and villages that embrace relational health and collaborate to meet the essential needs of families will yield positive developmental outcomes in health, education, and economic productivity. But villages are made of citizens, who must be educated, engaged, and empowered to ensure that their village is embracing relational health. Empowered citizens enhance their own lives, the lives of others, and the life of their community.

References

1. Espelage DL. Leveraging school-based research to inform bullying prevention and policy. *Am Psychol.* 2016;71(8):768–775
2. Espelage DL. Taking peer victimization research to the next level: complex interactions among genes, teacher attitudes/behaviors, peer ecologies, & classroom characteristics. *J Abnorm Child Psychol.* 2015;43(1):77–80
3. Sandy Hook Promise. Spread our message. http://www.sandyhookpromise.org/share_our_message. Accessed February 28, 2018
4. Sandy Hook Promise. Start with hello: promoting social inclusion and community connectedness. https://d3n8a8pro7vhmx.cloudfront.net/promise/pages/96/attachments/original/1442958562/Start_With_Hello.pdf?1442958562. Accessed February 28, 2018
5. Messing JT, Campbell J, Wilson JS, Brown S, Patchell B, Shall C. Police departments' use of the Lethality Assessment Program: a quasi-experimental evaluation. https://www.ncjrs.gov/pdffiles1/nij/grants/247456.pdf. Published March 31, 2014. Accessed February 28, 2018
6. Curran K, Drust B, Murphy R, Pringle A, Richardson D. The challenge and impact of engaging hard-to-reach populations in regular physical activity and health behaviours: an examination of an English Premier League 'Football in the Community' men's health programme. *Public Health.* 2016;135:14–22

7. City of Bloomington, MN. Adult sports and leagues. BloomingtonMN.gov Web site. https://www.bloomingtonmn.gov/pr/adult-sports-and-leagues. Accessed February 28, 2018

8. Paradis HA, Sandler M, Manly JT, Valentine L. Building healthy children: evidence-based home visitation integrated with pediatric medical homes. *Pediatrics.* 2013;132(Suppl 2):S174–S179

9. Garner AS. Home visiting and the biology of toxic stress: opportunities to address early childhood adversity. *Pediatrics.* 2013;132(Suppl 2):S65–S73

10. Chen L, Crockett AH, Covington-Kolb S, Heberlein E, Zhang L, Sun X. Centering and Racial Disparities (CRADLE study): rationale and design of a randomized controlled trial of CenteringPregnancy and birth outcomes. *BMC Pregnancy Childbirth.* 2017;17(1):118

11. Kania-Richmond A, Hetherington E, McNeil D, Bayrampour H, Tough S, Metcalfe A. The impact of introducing Centering Pregnancy in a community health setting: a qualitative study of experiences and perspectives of health center clinical and support staff. *Matern Child Health J.* 2017;21(6):1327–1335

12. Youth Challenge. History. http://www.youthchallengesports.com/Main/Blank.aspx. Accessed February 28, 2018

13. Ginsburg KR, Jablow MM. *Building Resilience in Children and Teens: Giving Kids Roots and Wings.* 3rd ed. Elk Grove Village, IL: American Academy of Pediatrics; 2015

14. Morrow-Howell N. Volunteering in later life: research frontiers. *J Gerontol B Psychol Sci Soc Sci.* 2010;65(4):461–469

15. Tang F, Choi E, Morrow-Howell N. Organizational support and volunteering benefits for older adults. *Gerontologist.* 2010;50(5):603–612

16. Samson A, Lavigne RM, MacPherson P. Self-fulfillment despite barriers: volunteer work of people living with HIV. *AIDS Care.* 2009;21(11):1425–1431

17. Bal MI, Sattoe JN, van Schaardenburgh NR, Floothuis MC, Roebroeck ME, Miedema HS. A vocational rehabilitation intervention for young adults with physical disabilities: participants' perception of beneficial attributes. *Child Care Health Dev.* 2017;43(1):114–125

18. Orth U, Maes J, Schmitt M. Self-esteem development across the life span: a longitudinal study with a large sample from Germany. *Dev Psychol.* 2015;51(2):248–259

19. Nelson SE, Gray HM, Maurice IR, Shaffer HJ. Moving ahead: evaluation of a work-skills training program for homeless adults. *Community Ment Health J.* 2012;48(6):711–722

20. Alliance for Strong Families and Communities. http://alliance1.org. Accessed February 28, 2018

21. United Way. https://www.unitedway.org. Accessed February 28, 2018

22. Kristof ND, WuDunn S. *A Path Appears: Transforming Lives, Creating Opportunity.* New York, NY: Alfred A. Knopf; 2014

23. Kristof N. From South Sudan to Yale. *The New York Times.* March 28, 2012. http://www.nytimes.com/2012/03/29/opinion/kristof-from-south-sudan-to-yale.html. Accessed February 28, 2018

24. Heckman JJ. Build a scaffolding of support. A comprehensive approach to human capital development pays off. *The Heckman Equation.* https://heckmanequation.org/assets/2017/01/F_Heckman_ScaffoldingSupport_0527215.pdf. Accessed February 28, 2018

25. Hawkins JD, Oesterle S, Brown EC, Abbott RD, Catalano RF. Youth problem behaviors 8 years after implementing the Communities That Care prevention system: a community-randomized trial. *JAMA Pediatr.* 2014;168(2):122–129

26. Rhew IC, Brown EC, Hawkins JD, Briney JS. Sustained effects of the Communities That Care system on prevention service system transformation. *Am J Public Health.* 2013;103(3):529–535

27. Hawkins JD, Catalano RF. *Communities That Care Prevention Strategies Guide.* 2004 ed. South Deerfield, MA: Channing Bete Co; 2004

28. Arthur MW, Hawkins JD, Pollard JA, Catalano RF, Baglioni AJ Jr. Measuring risk and protective factors for substance use, delinquency, and other adolescent problem behaviors. The Communities That Care Youth Survey. *Eval Rev.* 2002;26(6):575–601

29. Hawkins JD, Catalano RF, Kosterman R, Abbott R, Hill KG. Preventing adolescent health-risk behaviors by strengthening protection during childhood. *Arch Pediatr Adolesc Med.* 1999;153(3):226–234

30. Feldman HM. Reflections from a member of the AAP committee that prepared "Guidance for Effective Discipline." *Pediatrics.* 2016;138(6):e20162741

31. American Academy of Pediatrics Committee on Psychosocial Aspects of Child and Family Health. Guidance for effective discipline. *Pediatrics.* 1998;101(4):723–728

32. Zebel S, Schreurs W, Ufkes EG. Crime seriousness and participation in restorative justice: the role of time elapsed since the offense. *Law Hum Behav.* 2017;41(4):385–397

33. Ahlin EM, Gibbs JC, Kavanaugh PR, Lee J. Support for restorative justice in a sample of U.S. university students. *Int J Offender Ther Comp Criminol.* 2017;61(2):229–245

34. Riedl K, Jensen K, Call J, Tomasello M. Restorative justice in children. *Curr Biol.* 2015;25(13):1731–1735

35. Wenzel M, Okimoto TG, Feather NT, Platow MJ. Retributive and restorative justice. *Law Hum Behav.* 2008;32(5):375–389

36. Greene RW. *Lost at School: Why Our Kids with Behavioral Challenges Are Falling Through the Cracks and How We Can Help Them.* Rev ed. New York, NY: Scribner; 2014

37. Greene RW. *The Explosive Child: A New Approach for Understanding and Parenting Easily Frustrated, Chronically Inflexible Children.* Rev ed. New York, NY: Harper; 2014

38. Greene RW. *Raising Human Beings: Creating a Collaborative Partnership with Your Child.* New York, NY: Scribner; 2016

39. Saul RA. *My Children's Children: Raising Young Citizens in the Age of Columbine.* CreateSpace Independent Publishing Platform; 2013

40. Pronk TM, Karremans JC, Overbeek G, Vermulst AA, Wigboldus DH. What it takes to forgive: when and why executive functioning facilitates forgiveness. *J Pers Soc Psychol.* 2010;98(1):119–131

41. Horwitz L. The capacity to forgive: intrapsychic and developmental perspectives. *J Am Psychoanal Assoc.* 2005;53(2):485–511

42. Akhtar S. Forgiveness: origins, dynamics, psychopathology, and technical relevance. *Psychoanal Q.* 2002;71(2):175–212

43. Davis RM. Achieving racial harmony for the benefit of patients and communities: contrition, reconciliation, and collaboration. *JAMA.* 2008;300(3):323–325

44. Watt H. Doctor's group plans apology for racism: AMA once barred black physicians. *Washington Post.* July 10, 2008. http://www.myersfoundation.net/news4.html. Accessed February 28, 2018

45. Putnam RD. *Our Kids: The American Dream in Crisis.* New York, NY: Simon & Schuster; 2015

46. Putnam RD. *Bowling Alone: The Collapse and Revival of American Community.* New York, NY: Simon & Schuster; 2001

47. Johnson SL, Wibbels E, Wilkinson R. Economic inequality is related to cross-national prevalence of psychotic symptoms. *Soc Psychiatry Psychiatr Epidemiol.* 2015;50(12):1799–1807

48. Pickett KE, Wilkinson RG. The ethical and policy implications of research on income inequality and child well-being. *Pediatrics.* 2015;135(Suppl 2):S39–S47

49. Nowatzki NR. Wealth inequality and health: a political economy perspective. *Int J Health Serv.* 2012;42(3):403–424

50. Biggs B, King L, Basu S, Stuckler D. Is wealthier always healthier? The impact of national income level, inequality, and poverty on public health in Latin America. *Soc Sci Med.* 2010;71(2):266–273

51. Wilkinson R, Pickett K. *The Spirit Level: Why Greater Equality Makes Societies Stronger.* New York, NY: Bloomsbury Press; 2010

Chapter 9

The Role of Pediatric Care

· ·

Nobody cares how much you know,
until they know how much you care.

— *Theodore Roosevelt[1]*

· ·

The ecobiodevelopmental (EBD) model argues that investments in the early childhood ecology will improve life course trajectories because early childhood experiences, both affiliative and adverse, are biologically embedded and influence educational, health, and economic outcomes for decades to come. In the previous 3 chapters, we discussed the implications of this model for children, their families, and their communities. In this chapter, we will discuss the implications of the EBD model for pediatricians and other pediatric health care professionals (pediatric clinicians) and the care that they provide through family-centered pediatric medical homes (FCPMHs). Although this chapter might seem somewhat less relevant for readers who are not pediatricians, pediatric trainees, or medical students, the overarching theme holds true for all professionals who interact with young families: let them know how much you care before trying to share how much you know.

A Transformational Vision and Mission

The EBD model forces the entire pediatric community to embrace a much broader vision and mission.[2] The care that pediatricians provide cannot focus narrowly on infant and child development; it must lay the very foundations for healthy trajectories throughout the life course. The care that pediatricians provide cannot only be about the children; it must also be about their families, their communities, and the entire ecology within which those children develop. The care that pediatricians provide cannot only be about physical health; it must also be about relational health and surrounding young children with safe, stable, and nurturing relationships. Perhaps most importantly, the care pediatricians provide can no longer focus narrowly on acute or chronic care; it must reclaim wellness care as an integral component of what pediatricians do. As this vision of pediatric care expands, so does its mission to support parents, caregivers, and communities as they nurture their children's development. The implications of the EBD model for the practice of pediatrics are nothing short of transformational.[3,4]

Translating the science behind the EBD model into clinical practice will demand that the entire pediatric community, from primary care pediatric clinicians to chief executive officers of health care systems, embrace this broader vision and mission. The advances in basic developmental science discussed in Part 1 affect every aspect of pediatric care, from the way pediatric clinicians prioritize their clinical efforts, to the way researchers frame their research, to the way educators train the next generation of pediatricians, to the way the entire pediatric community advocates for young children and their families.[2] This chapter will briefly discuss how the EBD model informs each of the following important elements of pediatric care: clinical care, research, education, and advocacy.

Clinical Care

Reclaiming Wellness Care

Although well-child (health supervision) visits and prevention efforts have long been integral elements of pediatric care,[5,6] much of the contemporary interest in primary care medicine has focused on decreasing the costs of chronic conditions and preventing hospital readmissions through medical homes.[7,8] This concept of the medical home has recently been adopted by other fields of medicine, but its origin was in pediatrics, and its original objective was to coordinate care for children with special health care needs. From a public health perspective, *chronic care* is an example of tertiary prevention because it focuses on partnering with patients, their families, and their community resources to prevent the progression of an identified disease state (eg, asthma). *Acute care*, on the other hand, is more akin to secondary prevention and is focused on the early detection and initial stabilization of disease. Although the costly services provided in emergency departments are one example of acute care, retail- and school-based clinics increasingly provide acute care through less expensive, nonphysician professionals. The epitome of primary prevention, meanwhile, is *wellness care*, which is focused on partnering with patients, their families, and their community resources to proactively build healthy and resilient children.

Table 9-1 compares the essential elements of these 3 different types of pediatric care. Both wellness and chronic care require the collection and

Table 9-1. A Comparison of 3 Different Types of Pediatric Care

	Wellness Care	Acute (Sick) Care	Chronic (Specialty) Care
Type of Prevention	Primary	Secondary	Tertiary
Population	Universal	Selective or targeted (those who are symptomatic)	Indicated (those who are diagnosed)
Primary Objective	To promote wellness to avoid the occurrence of disease	To diagnose and treat disease in its early stages—before it causes significant morbidity or mortality	To reduce negative effects of known disease by restoring function and reducing disease-related complications
Essential Elements	• Promoting wellness • Actively building foundational skills (anticipatory guidance that encourages skill formation) • Ecobiodevelopmental *surveillance/screening for strengths and risk factors* • Immunizations	• Early identification and diagnosis of disease • Initial treatment or stabilization of disease • Initial disease education and explanation of the treatment plan • Planning for follow-up/communication with the medical home	• Ongoing disease education and management • Minimizing disease progression • *Promoting strengths and minimizing risk factors*
Example Resources	• Bright Futures • Connected Kids • Reach Out and Read	• BLS, PALS, or NALS • Algorithms for diagnosis/treatment	• Health supervision for Down (trisomy 21) syndrome, asthma, diabetes mellitus

(continued)

Table 9-1. A Comparison of 3 Different Types of Pediatric Care (*continued*)

	Wellness Care	Acute (Sick) Care	Chronic (Specialty) Care
Possible Venues	• *Medical homes* • *School-based health clinics* • Urgent care/retail-based clinics	• Emergency departments • Urgent care/retail-based clinics • Medical homes • School-based health clinics	• *Medical homes* • Specialty care clinics • *School-based health clinics*
Importance of Continuity (Therapeutic Relationship)	*Extremely important: A therapeutic relationship is essential.*	Somewhat important: A therapeutic partnership is helpful.	*Extremely important: A therapeutic relationship is essential.*
Importance of Context (Social and Family Histories)	*Extremely important: A deep understanding of context is essential.*	Somewhat important: An understanding of context is helpful.	*Extremely important: A deep understanding of context is essential.*
Amenable to Algorithms	*Less amenable: Care plans must be personalized.*	Extremely amenable: Care plans are often generalizable.	*Less amenable: Care plans must be personalized.*
Addressed in Training	*Limited training opportunities*	Extensive training opportunities	*Limited training opportunities*
Incentivized Through Payment	*Minimal incentives (lower patient volumes; bundling of services)*	Major incentives (larger patient volumes; billing for procedures)	*Minimal incentives (lower patient volumes; bundling of services)*
Long-term Returns on Initial Investment	Large (eg, immunizations)	Variable (depends on diagnosis/acuity)	Moderate (eg, well-controlled diabetes mellitus)

Abbreviations: BLS, basic life support; NALS, neonatal advanced life support; PALS, pediatric advanced life support.

The concept of the *medical home* grew from the need to provide specialty care to children with chronic conditions. The elements and attributes that chronic specialty care shares with wellness care are highlighted in *italics*.

integration of a wide array of information, including family and social history and the surveillance of the child's and family's strengths and risk factors. Wellness and chronic care are, therefore, less amenable to straightforward algorithms. They also receive less attention in most training programs, despite their ability to provide significant returns on investment over a longer term. Wellness and chronic care are currently not as incentivized in the health care system as acute care because they require fewer procedures and more time to build a therapeutic relationship. To be done well, and not just perfunctorily, both wellness and chronic care require health care professionals who excel at forming therapeutic relationships and integrating a wide array of information into care plans that are unique and personalized for an individual child and his or her specific needs.

The Centrality of Therapeutic Relationships

Although a therapeutic relationship might facilitate the delivery of acute care (eg, consenting to an emergent surgical procedure), it is absolutely essential for the delivery of wellness and chronic care. To prevent the *onset* of a disease (primary prevention) or the *progression* of a disease over time (tertiary prevention), pediatricians must partner with the child, the family, and other caregivers (eg, teachers, coaches) to strengthen health-promoting behaviors, minimize health risks, and, simply, promote change. In this context, the relationship between the pediatrician and the caregivers *is* the therapeutic intervention because it is the vehicle that allows the pediatric clinician to intervene on behalf of the child. Without trusting, respectful, therapeutic relationships, primary care pediatricians and all their well-intentioned advice are but "noisy gongs and clanging cymbals"[9] because nobody is actually listening to them. In the words of Theodore Roosevelt, "Nobody cares how much you know, until they know how much you care."[1] This must become the mantra for all pediatric clinicians who aim to reclaim wellness care and strive to support parents, caregivers, and communities as they nurture their children's development.[2] In the end, families and the patients themselves are the ultimate agents of change. For pediatricians to have an effect on long-term outcomes, we must embrace the centrality of therapeutic relationships and reclaim childhood wellness care as an integral element of pediatric care and a requisite foundation for lifelong health and prosperity.

A Focus on Building Relational Health

A major implication of the EBD model is that safe, stable, and nurturing relationships are the antidote for childhood adversity and toxic stress. Translating this understanding into clinical practice requires that pediatricians (and the

FCPMHs that they direct) remain focused on the child's and family's relational health. As discussed in previous chapters, a public health approach to relational health would include at least 3 elements: *repairing relational health* when it has become strained; *identifying and eliminating potential barriers to relational health;* and actively *promoting relational health in a universal manner* (see Figure 6-1). To have an effect, FCPMHs must embrace each of these levels because all will be necessary and none alone will be sufficient to improve relational health and/or developmental outcomes at the population level.

To illustrate how the EBD model and a steady focus on relational health might transform the way pediatric clinicians approach clinical care, we will first provide and discuss a few hypothetical case vignettes. Although these cases are entirely fictional, they reflect concerns that confront pediatric clinicians every day, challenging the way we prioritize and frame what we do. Recall that a development-informed approach asks not "What is wrong with you?" or "How can I fix you?" but "What has happened (or is happening) to you?" and "How can I better understand you?" By first focusing on relational health (the clinician-parent relationship and the parent-child dyad), pediatric clinicians are better positioned to treat the sick and build the well. But working on relationships is a fundamentally different operation than following clinical guidelines. The ambiguity of not knowing precisely what to say or how others might respond seems fraught with peril when compared with straightforward algorithms for decision-making. In fact, the comments and responses of the clinicians in these cases are not intended to represent the gold-standard or only way to approach these situations. Rather, they are provided as examples of how a focus on relational health changes the way pediatric clinicians approach clinical care.

Repairing Relational Health: A Clinical Vignette

A mom presents with her 2-year-old son for an ear check. "He's been more awful than usual," she says. "He's crying all the time, not sleeping, not eating, and definitely not listening." On examination, you confirm that he does indeed have a right ear infection. After checking for drug allergies and dutifully prescribing amoxicillin, you have just begun to explain your treatment plan when the child bolts out of the room and runs down the hall. Mom gives chase and returns to the room, dragging the screaming child in a manner that makes you worry about nursemaid elbow. Before you can examine the child's elbow, Mom yells angrily, "Stop being so evil!" and briskly spanks him on the buttocks.

You want nothing more than to simply review the treatment plan for the ear infection and move on to the next patient. But your grounding in the EBD model allows you to see that the ear infection is not the biggest threat to this child's long-term health. So, after explaining the treatment for the ear infection and confirming that the child does not have a dislocated elbow, you take a deep breath and ask Mom, "Do you really think that your son is evil?"

You are heartbroken when she glibly replies, "Absolutely. He wants nothing more than to hit me and run away from me."

You reply, "I have no doubt that he is a handful, and it sounds like you are pretty frustrated. I frequently see children and moms struggle at this age when there is a mismatch between our expectations and the child's abilities. My experience is that a child's behavior is often his way of trying to have his needs met. For example, he might not be running away or hitting you because he does not like you, as you have suggested. He might be doing that because he knows it will get your attention and you will chase him. I'm no expert in this subject, but there are some counselors in the area that are very good at teaching moms and their kids how to better understand each other. Would you be interested in learning some less stressful ways to help him behave?"

Much to your relief, she agrees, and you provide the name and number of a local therapist who specializes in parent-child interaction therapy (PCIT). You dutifully note this referral in the chart so you can follow up in the future. If she had refused the referral (or if she does not complete the referral on follow-up), you might consider mentioning that "corporal punishment is associated with poor long-term outcomes, like being more aggressive when older, and I know you don't want that for your son. So please call the office if and when you are ready to learn about some alternative forms of discipline that might be more effective and less stressful for both of you."

Repairing Relational Health: A Discussion

This first case highlights the clinician pivoting from a biomedical model (an ear infection is the problem and amoxicillin is the fix) to an EBD model (the strained parent-child relationship is the biggest threat to this child's life course, so I need to understand the barriers). Clearly, when a mother believes that her son is evil, there has been a major breach in the dyadic relationship, and that breach bodes poorly for the son's future health, academic success, and economic productivity.

Most parents want their children to thrive. But when parents (and children!) are in survival mode, they may revert to quick fixes or behaviors that they have found to be effective in the past. Over time, these behaviors (eg, yelling, berating, spanking) might strain the dyadic relationship, making the learning of new behaviors more difficult for both generations. Consequently, interventions like PCIT, Attachment and Biobehavioral Catch-up (ABC), and child-parent psychotherapy (CPP) repair the dyadic relationship and use that safe, stable, and nurturing relationship to build new skills in a 2-generational manner. A referral to this sort of intervention is merited whenever the clinician suspects a breach in the dyadic relationship, and a mother calling her son evil would most certainly qualify.

Witnessing the use of corporal punishment does not necessarily mean the dyadic relationship has been irreparably harmed, but it is certainly a red flag. Unfortunately, corporal punishment is a common practice.[10-12] Although it may succeed in altering a child's behavior in the short term, corporal punishment is known to be less effective than other forms of discipline and is associated with more aggression over time.[12-18] Although many parents would prefer not to spank their children, they often feel they have no other options or that spanking is the right thing to do.[10,19,20] Moreover, spanking is often done when the parent or caregiver is angry, teaching young children that "it is OK to hit when you are upset."[21]

More importantly for pediatric clinicians grounded in the EBD model, corporal punishment is a major threat to relational health. Although not all parents who engage in corporal punishment will have a poor relationship with their children, many parents who do have poor relationships with their children will use corporal punishment.[22-24] Recall, however, that *discipline* means to teach, and neuroscience tells us that young children do not learn complex lessons well when they are scared. If a child's behavior is a means of communicating an unfulfilled need (eg, "I need attention and connection"; "I need stimulation and opportunities to build esteem"), and the parent/caregiver role is to teach the child more adaptive ways to have that need met, there can be no role for corporal punishment because it will interfere with the child's ability to learn those more adaptive behaviors. If safe, stable, and nurturing relationships and relational health are the antidotes to toxic stress, parents and caregivers interested in promoting optimal early brain and child development need to make certain their children feel safe, first, foremost, and always.

One concept worth mentioning here is the fundamental difference between fear and respect. Some pro–corporal punishment advocates have argued that children must fear the parent to respect the parent.[25] But many people respect leaders like the Pope, Gandhi, and Martin Luther King Jr, while being unlikely to fear them. True respect is earned, not forced out of fear. If young children fear anything, it is the loss of the connection and understanding that they receive from their parents and caregivers. But time out from that connection and understanding is only effective if relational health is the norm and there is plenty of time in.

Unfortunately, the use of corporal punishment is but one of many red flags for poor relational health that pediatric clinicians need to recognize.[22] In fact, many of the conflicts that parents and caregivers have with young children can be, at least in part, traced back to the relational health of the parent/ caregiver-child dyad. Poor emotion regulation (eg, being fussy), poor feeding, poor sleeping, and difficulties with stranger anxiety, separation anxiety, and sensory issues are all associated with impaired attachments and disruptions in the dyadic relationship.[26–43] That said, not all children with these concerns have poor relational health with their caregivers, as there is a wide degree of variability in the typical temperaments of young children. Moreover, some may argue about which came first, poor relational health leading to disruptive behaviors or disruptive behaviors leading to poor relational health. But arguing over which came first is a moot point because the relationship is the foundation; it is the vital, first step forward in teaching the child more adaptive behaviors. This is why many developmental and behavioral pediatricians are taught to begin their interventions by challenging the parents to "catch them being good." Encouragement and praise, particularly if given for efforts and not necessarily outcomes, is an effective way of beginning to heal broken dyads.[44–49] In addition to developmental and behavioral pediatricians, therapists with specialized training in PCIT,[50–53] CPP,[54–56] and ABC[57–60] are well positioned to work with families to repair relational health and set the stage for learning more adaptive behaviors.

Identifying Potential Barriers to Relational Health: A Case Vignette

A 7-year-old presents for his first well-child check with you. His father reports that they have recently moved into the area from out of state. As you quickly scan the boy's old medical records, you notice that, although he has been relatively healthy and his immunizations are up-to-date, his body mass index has recently skyrocketed to above the 99th percentile for his age. You also note that his previous pediatrician called child and family services because she was concerned that his mother was neglecting him. When you ask Dad about those concerns, he states that he was not caring for his son at that time; he and the child's mother separated when the son was younger than 1 year and Mom struggled with depression and substance abuse before overdosing on heroin last year. Dad was then given custody, and he decided to move to a new state with the hope of giving his son a fresh start.

As always, you begin by asking Dad if he had any concerns about his son. Dad flatly denies any concerns, saying that, although his son has been through a lot, he did well in first grade and seemed to make a lot of new friends at school. He also proudly reports that his son was "really small when I got him, but he's doing well now."

Because you are concerned about the child's obesity, you ask dad about his diet. Dad reports that he is currently working 2 part-time jobs, which allows him to put his son on the bus in the morning and to be at home when he gets off the bus in the afternoon. Because Dad's evening job is at a fast-food restaurant, his son usually gets his dinner there. When you ask about snacks between meals, Dad says, "I tend to give him whatever he wants because he has been through so much."

When you ask the son what he likes to eat, he says, "Cookies, chips, and French fries."

You also ask about opportunities for exercise. Dad reports that he offered to sign his son up for soccer, but his son refused because it requires "too much running" and he would much rather play video games. When you ask Dad if he is concerned that his son is so large, he says, "Nope. When I was his age I was bullied every day at school. But I was a shrimp, so my feeling is that the bigger he is, the better."

You quickly realize that there is more work to be done than can be accomplished in a one visit, so you begin to prioritize a treatment plan that is entirely dependent on the father returning with his son for follow-up appointments. You focus on building a rapport with Dad, learning more about his upbringing as a child and his more recent struggles as a single parent. You congratulate him for giving his son a fresh start and for finding ways to be with him as much as possible. You also let him know that you are concerned about his son's weight because, over time, this could become a real threat to his health and longevity. You affirm that Dad wants to do right by his son, and you understand his desire to be responsive to his son's calls for food and ensure that his son is not bullied.

As a first step, you ask Dad if he thinks his son's eating and love of video games are somehow related to his son's adversity as a young child. When Dad looks at you quizzically, you share that it is not uncommon for kids who have experienced significant adversity as a child to look for ways to cope with ongoing stress or worry. You explain that his son may not remember the adversity, but his body remembers, and it may always be in flight or fight mode. As a consequence, kids are often looking for ways to turn off that anxious or uneasy feeling, and 2 very effective ways of turning off stress are eating and escaping into a very predictable and less scary electronic universe. By explaining these behaviors as adaptations to adversity, you are not blaming the father or the son, and you are laying the groundwork for a potential way forward: building more adaptive coping styles and healthy distractions.

As you complete your physical examination, you ask the son to think about what his passions are. "What are the things that you would do all day long if given the chance?" After he predictably answers "Minecraft," you ask what he would love to do all day that is not electronic. Now the son looks at you quizzically! So you ask about reading, drawing, toys, or sports. Dad then chimes in that he likes sports but is not a big fan of competition. So you suggest individual sports, like running, swimming, dancing, or learning a martial art. The son is thrilled at the idea of becoming a real-life ninja, so you give Dad some information about a free, introductory tae kwon do class at the local recreation center. You suggest to Dad that this might be a good way to learn self-defense and get some exercise. You also explain to Dad that kids who are overweight are targets for bullying, just like kids who are underweight. So, if we want to minimize additional trauma for his son, we may want to work on ways for him to lose some weight or simply maintain his weight as he grows into it. Dad affirms that he really wants to minimize additional trauma for his son, and he agrees to come back to the office in the next month or so to brainstorm about other ways to lose weight and build healthy coping skills. You close the visit by mentioning that there are also biological reasons that kids rapidly gain weight, like type 2 diabetes or hypothyroidism, so you really need to see him back in the next few weeks.

At future visits you rule out diabetes and thyroid disease, and you use motivational interviewing techniques to assess their interest and ideas on how to access healthier foods, limit screen time, and get more exercise. In particular, you focus on their relationship and ways they might work together as a team. For example, the child might be more inclined to continue with the tae kwon do classes if Dad takes them as well. Or Dad might agree to spend 20 minutes each night playing a video game *with* his son if the son agrees to then turn off the video games for the rest of the evening. With Dad's assistance and attention, the child might then develop other, more adaptive interests, like checkers, chess, reading, practicing his tae kwon do forms, or learning a new magic trick. Shared experiences strengthen the bond and build new, more adaptive skills at the same time.

Identifying Potential Barriers to Relational Health: A Discussion

This second case study illustrates the ability of the EBD model to make sense of complex, multifactorial phenomena (eg, adverse childhood experiences [ACEs], obesity, screen time, good-enough parenting) that are frequently interrelated. It also highlights the importance of identifying and addressing potential barriers to relational health.

Briefly consider the traditional problem list ("What is wrong with you?") and treatments ("How I can fix you?") that might result from this visit if the pediatric clinician used a biomedical or biopsychosocial model.

1. Obesity: Rule out organic etiologies.
2. Excessive screen time: Counsel on limiting screen time.
3. Sedentary lifestyle: Counsel on getting more exercise.
4. Poor diet: Refer to nutritionist.
5. An overly indulgent father: Counsel on how to set limits and manage conflict.
6. Histories of adversity (both son and father): Refer to different therapists for the son and father.

Remember, this is the first visit that this child and father are having with you. This father is bending over backwards to do right by his son, and he is justifiably proud for stepping up to care for him. If he senses that you believe he is doing anything *wrong* or that he is in any way *not* being a good-enough parent, you may not see him ever again.

So how do you proceed? First, apply the EBD model to the child. We could start with his significant adversity. Even with the little information provided, we already know the son's ACE score is at least 4 (maternal depression, household substance abuse, parental separation, and physical neglect). Then briefly consider the biological and developmental outcomes that could be associated with this adversity. These include a chronic flight or fight response; higher or dysregulated cortisol levels; a larger, more potent amygdala; and a relatively less potent prefrontal cortex. In brief, this child is more likely to be in survival mode than relational mode (see Figure 4-3). He may also adopt behaviors (eg, overeating, escaping into the electronic universe, avoiding others, socially withdrawing) that transiently allow him to cope with this chronic stress (behavioral allostasis). When viewed from this EBD perspective, we cannot reasonably ask the son to give up his current coping mechanisms (emotional eating and screen time) unless we give him some alternatives! Hence, our first objective is to assist him in building some healthier coping techniques, like exercise (eg, sports, dancing, walking a pet), creative arts (eg, coloring, crafts, building toys), or mental gymnastics (eg, jigsaw puzzles, Rush Hour, Mastermind). But to effectively build those new skills, we need parents, teachers, coaches, pediatricians, and other adults to first develop a safe, stable, and nurturing relationship with the child.

Also apply the EBD model to the father. He experienced at least one form of childhood adversity: being bullied. Because he attributes this to his small size, he does not recognize the health-harming consequences of obesity. At this point (the initial visit), we know little else about the father, but in follow-up visits we will explore more about his childhood and the lessons that he does (and does not) want to repeat with his son. For example, if the father's father never provided materially for him, the father may see his principal role as being the provider of material goods. This might explain the father's drive to manage 2 jobs. But if the father's father never taught him how to be an engaged (stable) and encouraging (nurturing) adult, developing a safe, stable, and nurturing relationship with his son might prove to be difficult.

Obesity is a complex, multifactorial disease process that can no longer be understood simply in terms of calories eaten and burned.[61–66] As in this vignette, obesity is often inextricably linked to economic status and social-emotional factors.[67–72] For example, poverty can result in food insecurity, which is, paradoxically, associated with obesity.[73–77] Poverty can also limit the father's opportunities to unwind, engage, and actually play with his son.[78] Such shared moments are important because they strengthen their relationship, decrease their physiologic stress, and allow for the father to assist the child in building new skills.

But there are other social-emotional factors at play here as well. The father is aware of the adversity that his son has had to bear in his short life. But instead of assisting his son in learning healthy ways to cope, he has chosen to indulge his son's most primal coping mechanisms: overeating and escaping into the electronic universe. Finally, the father may also be dealing with his own demons. By attributing the ACEs from his own childhood to his size at the time (and not to the social ineptitude of the bullies), he is trying to protect his son by giving him mass, instead of healthy coping skills. As pediatricians, we know that being obese makes the son more likely to be bullied,[79–82] but Dad's interpretation of his own childhood adversity tells him otherwise.

Discussions about obesity are hard enough when simply focusing on the physiology, and those discussions about nutrition, exercise, screen time, and sleep are important ones to have with families. But pediatric clinicians grounded in the EBD model recognize that discussions about the barriers to relational health, while perhaps more sensitive and difficult, are nevertheless even more critical because they lay the foundation for insight, healing, and the learning of new behaviors. To the clinician grounded in the EBD model, all the so-called social determinants of health (eg, parental depression, parental substance abuse, parental separation or divorce, domestic violence, poverty, food insecurity, neighborhood violence) are potential barriers to the safe, stable, and nurturing relationships and relational health that buffer young children from all forms of adversity. That is not to say that the social determinants of health make it impossible for children to develop safe, stable, and nurturing relationships, but they do make relational health more difficult.

A public health approach to obesity and other diseases associated with behavioral allostasis (see discussion on the Big 5 in Chapter 1) will require pediatric clinicians to identify and address child-, family-, and community-level barriers to relational health. Although pediatricians have long acknowledged the tremendous effect of the social determinants of health on a child's development and life course trajectory, actually identifying these family- and community-level risk factors will require a different sort of screening. Developmental and disease screening often use standardized tools (with cutoffs, sensitivities, and specificities) that are designed to be administered identically to many different patients and families. But the identification of family- and community-level concerns is much more akin to a very personal disclosure. If not done within the context of a trusting and mutually respectful therapeutic relationship, parental disclosures of unemployment, poverty, food insecurity, depression, or their own childhood adversities could potentially alienate already disenfranchised families and, at least theoretically, do more damage than good.[83]

Poverty has a pervasive influence that can affect even the most secure relationships because it is hard for parents and children to be in relational mode and mindful of others when they are in survival mode. Poverty not only affects the genome[84,85] and brain[86,87] of the developing child; it also has long-term effects on other organ systems. Many disorders of adulthood (eg, obesity, hypertension, diabetes, heart disease) are expressed more frequently in individuals exposed to the toxic stress responses triggered by poverty.[88–92] As previously discussed, these so-called adult-onset disorders are actually adult-*manifest* disorders caused, at least in part, by childhood experiences.

Finally, poverty and economic disparities harm not only the individuals living in poverty but their entire community. Recall that data from the Organisation for Economic Co-operation and Development, the World Bank, and others demonstrate that the wider the degree of economic disparity (as measured by the Gini coefficient), the worse everyone in that society fares—including the wealthy.[93–96] Poverty and economic inequities undermine social connectedness and relational health, making maladaptive behaviors like the Big 5 (see discussion on behavioral allostasis in Chapter 1) more common and the diseases associated with these behaviors (eg, obesity, smoking, substance abuse) harder to treat.

Recognizing the health-harming consequences of economic inequities, the American Academy of Pediatrics (AAP) issued a policy statement on poverty in 2016 (www.aap.org/poverty)[97] that noted the following foci for intervention: food insecurity, housing insecurity/homelessness, income insecurity, paid family leave, early childhood support, and economic and community development. All of these areas for intervention might seem disconnected from

Box 9-1. Tips for Pediatricians and Key Messages, American Academy of Pediatrics Poverty Initiative

Tip 1: Emphasize the connection between poverty and child health by focusing on poverty as a key determinant of child health.

Key messages
1. Linkage of poverty to higher rates of asthma and obesity, poor language development, increased infant mortality, and an increased risk of injuries
2. Linkage of poverty and toxic stress to chronic cardiovascular disease and immune and psychiatric (including behavioral) disorders

Tip 2: Talk about ways to address child poverty and improve the life course trajectory for children by highlighting policies and programs with proven social and economic benefits.

Key messages
1. Childhood poverty is a lifelong hardship with multiple health issues and limiting economic potential—preventable.
2. Poverty is a substantial economic drain for society ($500 billion/y in low productivity and poor health) with a great risk for crime and incarceration—preventable.
3. Healthy children need financially secure parents, so programs need to lift families out of poverty.

Derived from American Academy of Pediatrics Council on Community Pediatrics. Poverty and child health in the United States. *Pediatrics.* 2016;137(4):e20160339.

straightforward medical care, but health care professionals grounded in the EBD model will recognize them as being vital to the physical and relational health of children and their families. Box 9-1 lists the tips and key messages from the AAP poverty initiative.

Actively Promoting Relational Health: Case 1

While examining a 5-week-old during her 1-month well-child checkup, you elicit a social smile. The parents are thrilled that their daughter "likes you!" You affirm that social smiles (not just smiling for no reason, but smiling in response to a face) are indeed magical moments because parents are able to have more of a relationship with their child. You go on to explain that the ongoing dance between the parent and the child, the so-called serve and return, builds their bond as well as her brain. Social smiles are also a starting point for a discussion on discipline, in that *discipline* means to teach, not to punish. So, if every time their daughter smiles, a face appears and smiles back at her, she will keep smiling. Similarly, if every time she coos, a face appears and coos back at her, she will continue to coo. But if Mom is depressed or the parents are too busy to respond, she may quickly realize that the only way to get attention is to scream her head off. You encourage the parents to be responsive and to "catch her being good" because it is a lot easier, and a lot more fun, than trying to keep her from doing something they would rather she not do—like screaming.

Actively Promoting Relational Health: Case 2

When you enter the room for a 9-month well-child check, the infant sees your face and quickly turns to look at his mother. Because the mother is attuned to her son's attention, she smiles at her son, and he begins to relax. After briefly greeting everyone, you ask the mother if she noted what just happened. "When confronted with a stranger—me—your son quickly looked to you to see if I was a good guy or a threat. That is called *social referencing,* and it means that he is literally reading your face. Because you noted his concern and smiled back at him, he relaxed. But if you were distracted or appeared to be concerned about me or anything else, he may have started screaming due to stranger anxiety. The point here is that we think of language as only being spoken, but one of the first languages children understand is emotion. When children get older, we often encourage parents to watch what they say because they may hear their children say it as well. At this age, we encourage parents to watch what their faces are saying because children will likely share that emotion with them. You may not be angry with your son, but if you are stressed out due to work or angry at his sibling, he will read your face and feel your stress and anger. That doesn't mean that you should try to hide your emotions, because that could be even more confusing for him. But it is worth trying to temper your emotions because children are very sensitive to strong emotions at this age."

Actively Promoting Relational Health: A Discussion

Universal interventions to promote relational health are the foundation of a public health approach to support wellness. As Frederick Douglass once said, "It is easier to build strong children than to repair broken men."[98] But the current health care system is primarily focused on repairing broken men (tertiary care), and only occasionally do we go upstream to address risk factors (secondary care), let alone implement universal preventions (primary care).

The previous 2 case vignettes demonstrate a generalizable approach for promoting relational health in pediatric care: identify childhood developmental milestones, explain to parents why they are significant, and use them as examples of how parents can proactively build the dyadic dance with their children.[99] Smiling "conversations" lead to cooing conversations, which lead to the dyadic dance needed for the feeding of solid foods, which leads to emotional conversations and social referencing, which leads to receptive language skills and, eventually, expressive language skills. Relational health is all about the dance, the serve and return between the child and caregiver that builds bonds and brains at the same time.[100]

These examples also demonstrate that promoting the dyadic dance does not require a lot of additional time, but it may prevent disruptions in the dance from occurring in the first place. For example, a discussion about the social smile could also be an opportunity to address a mother's depression and her need to take care of herself so she is able to catch her infant being good and to smile back whenever those social smiles emerge. A discussion about social referencing could also be an opportunity to address parental screen time and the need for parents to put the phone away so they are able to engage with their child.[101]

Other universal interventions to promote relational health include Reach Out and Read[102,103] and developmentally appropriate play.[78,104] Although Reach Out and Read is frequently cited as an intervention to promote early literacy, its real power is its ability to promote relational health. In Reach Out and Read, the book becomes a concrete tool for promoting the dance and the shared attunement that comes from reading books together. Similarly, studies have shown that simply teaching parents how to engage in developmentally appropriate play decreases violence and increases academic achievement decades later.[104] Group well-child visits,[105–108] Healthy Steps,[109–111] and the Video Interaction Project[112–114] are other promising practices to promote relational health in a universal, proactive manner.

Final Thoughts on Clinical Care

The EBD model suggests that the way to prevent early childhood adversity and toxic stress from altering life course trajectories in a negative manner is to implement a public health approach to building relational health. At a minimum, this will require treatments (eg, PCIT, ABC, CPP) that repair strained relationships, strategies for identifying and addressing threats to relational health (eg, poverty, parental depression or substance abuse), and universal strategies to promote a healthy dyadic dance right from the start. All these will be necessary, and none of them alone will be sufficient.

Similarly, the inclusion of FCPMHs in this public health agenda will be absolutely necessary for its success, yet FCPMHs, in and of themselves, are insufficient to ensure success. To become development-informed and translate the EBD model into pediatric care, FCPMHs must embrace a 2-generation approach (help the parents to help the kids) and acknowledge the need for team-based care (eg, pediatricians, nurses, medical assistants, case managers, parenting counselors, developmental specialists, nutritionists, medicolegal consultants, speech therapists). No single health care professional, pediatrician or otherwise, can provide all the different levels of care or coordinate a family's care with a myriad of community resources. A major priority of the AAP Task Force on Pediatric Practice Change is payment reform because restructured payment models will be needed to make 2-generation and team-based care financially feasible for FCPMHs.

Finally, it has been proposed that there should be 3 primary objectives for nationwide health care reform; the so-called triple aims are higher quality care, lower cost, and higher patient satisfaction.[115,116] To date, however, only higher quality and lower costs have received a great deal of attention. Once health care reform begins to measure and track patient satisfaction, health care professionals who understand the EBD model, embrace the centrality of therapeutic relationships, and focus on building relational health are likely to fare well. Recently, family medicine practitioners have proposed a "quadruple aim" by adding a fourth objective: health care professional satisfaction.[117] It seems intuitive that health care professionals who are stuck in the old medical model of "What is wrong with you? I must fix it," are likely to be more frustrated and not as likely to experience professional satisfaction as those who have adopted the development-informed model of "What has happened to you? I am called to listen and to understand you."

A Call for Continued Research

Much of the broader pediatric community is not focused on the provision of direct clinical care but on pediatric research. The EBD model has important implications for how pediatric research is framed and prioritized.[2] As discussed in Chapter 2, the basic science of pediatrics is development, so more basic pediatric research needs to be framed within a broader life course perspective. Priority should be given to research with the potential of yielding additional insights into how early experiences are biologically embedded and influence learning, behavior, and health decades later. Moreover, minimally invasive, practice-friendly biomarkers of toxic stress responses (eg, specific methylation patterns, telomere length, patterns of brain connectivity) are needed to stratify risk and perhaps even to monitor the effectiveness of different interventions. Advances in quality improvement science will need to be mobilized as practices implement interventions, quantify their effect, and integrate them into the flow of clinical practice. Finally, and perhaps most importantly, we know that relational health is the secret sauce that protects children from adversity and toxic stress, but how do we go about objectively measuring relational health? Safe, stable, and nurturing relationships are the goal, but how do we quantify the degree to which relationships are safe, stable, or nurturing? Practice-friendly measures of shared attunement and emotional reciprocity are desperately needed to move pediatric research and pediatric clinical care to the next level.

Educating the Next Generation of Health Care Professionals

As discussed in Chapter 5, the EBD model has important implications for undergraduate medical education. All medical professionals, not only pediatricians, need to think developmentally to fully understand the childhood origins of adult-manifest disease. Recall that the ACE Study grew out of research on adult morbid obesity and that many of the patients who were most obese were unable to sustain their dramatic weight loss because obesity had become a mechanism for coping with their unresolved childhood adversity.[118] Understanding the link between ACEs and their obesity allowed these patients to heal from their past trauma and learn more adaptive ways to cope with their ongoing stress. Teaching medical students the advantages of the EBD model will encourage all medical professionals to think developmentally and to consider the childhood origins of adult-manifest disease. But the EBD model suggests even more dramatic changes for pediatric trainees.[2] Pediatric residents need additional training in developmental and behavioral pediatrics[119–121]; epigenetics, neuroscience, and toxic stress[122,123]; the capacity of safe, stable, and nurturing relationships and relational health to buffer adversity[100,124,125]; the provision of 2-generational and team-based care[126]; and the application of a public health approach[127,128] to complex and seemingly intractable problems like poverty, violence, and childhood adversity.

Advocacy Grounded in the Ecobiodevelopmental Model

The EBD model of disease and wellness suggests that for the health care system to improve outcomes and decrease costs, it needs to expand from a narrow focus on treating adult-manifest physical disease to include the promotion of relational health beginning at birth—if not before. But as we have seen, many of the barriers to relational health (eg, parental academic achievement and employment; parental depression or substance abuse; food insecurity; racism or social exclusion) fall outside the traditional role of pediatric care. As pediatricians continue to advocate for the wellness of their patients and families, they must also advocate for concerns that might seem outside their traditional sphere of influence—areas like educational policy, the accessibility and scope of social services, and strategies to improve economic productivity and minimize economic disparities. Clearly, the EBD model has important implications for public policy beyond the realm of health care, and these will be addressed in the next chapter.

But the EBD model also empowers pediatric clinicians with our own unique approach to collective advocacy. Ethicists might well argue that early investments in children and their families are the right thing to do ethically, but pediatricians are not ethicists. Economists might well argue that early investments in children and their families are the right thing to do economically, but pediatricians are not economists. The power of the EBD model is that it allows pediatricians to say confidently that early investments in children and their families are the right thing to do *biologically*, and pediatricians are acknowledged, respected, and trusted experts on child biology.

Conclusions

The EBD model explains how early childhood adversity and toxic stress affect child development and adult outcomes in a negative manner. But it also explains how safe, stable, and nurturing relationships and relational health can buffer children from adversity and toxic stress. Translating this science into clinical practice will be a monumental process, but the first steps include

1. Reclaiming wellness care as an integral element of pediatric care
2. Recognizing the centrality of therapeutic relationships
3. Repairing strained dyads as early as possible
4. Identifying and addressing barriers to relational health, including a wide array of social determinants of health
5. Promoting relational health in a universal manner by helping parents and caregivers to engage in developmentally appropriate versions of the dyadic dance

This translation of science into practice will also require sustained investments in research, changes in medical education and the training of new pediatricians, and a clear, biology-grounded focus in the way the pediatric community advocates for patients and their families.

References

1. Roosevelt T. BrainyQuote Web site. https://www.brainyquote.com/quotes/theodore_roosevelt_140484. Accessed March 1, 2018
2. Garner AS. Thinking developmentally: the next evolution in models of health. *J Dev Behav Pediatr.* 2016;37(7):579–584

3. Shonkoff JP, Garner AS; American Academy of Pediatrics Committee on Psychosocial Aspects of Child and Family Health; Committee on Early Childhood, Adoption, and Dependent Care; Section on Developmental and Behavioral Pediatrics. Technical report: the lifelong effects of early childhood adversity and toxic stress. *Pediatrics.* 2012;129(1):e232–e246

4. American Academy of Pediatrics Committee on Psychosocial Aspects of Child and Family Health; Committee on Early Childhood, Adoption, and Dependent Care; Section on Developmental and Behavioral Pediatrics. Policy statement: early childhood adversity, toxic stress, and the role of the pediatrician: translating developmental science into lifelong health. *Pediatrics.* 2012;129(1):e224–e231

5. American Academy of Pediatrics. *Dedicated to the Health of All Children.* Baker JP, Pearson HA, eds. Elk Grove Village, IL: American Academy of Pediatrics; 2005

6. Hagan JF, Shaw JS, Duncan PM, eds. *Bright Futures: Guidelines for Health Supervision of Infants, Children, and Adolescents.* 4th ed. Elk Grove Village, IL: American Academy of Pediatrics; 2017

7. Sia C, Tonniges TF, Osterhus E, Taba S. History of the medical home concept. *Pediatrics.* 2004;113(Suppl 4):1473–1478

8. Sia CC, Peter MI. Physician involvement strategies to promote the medical home. *Pediatrics.* 1990;85(1):128–130

9. 1 Corinthians 13:1. Bible Gateway Web site. https://www.biblegateway.com/passage/?search=1 Corinthians 13:1-2&version=RSV. Accessed March 1, 2018

10. Chiocca EM. American parents' attitudes and beliefs about corporal punishment: an integrative literature review. *J Pediatr Health Care.* 2017;31(3):372–383

11. Ryan RM, Kalil A, Ziol-Guest KM, Padilla C. Socioeconomic gaps in parents' discipline strategies from 1988 to 2011. *Pediatrics.* 2016;138(6):e20160720

12. Zolotor AJ. Corporal punishment. *Pediatr Clin North Am.* 2014;61(5):971–978

13. Thompson R, Kaczor K, Lorenz DJ, Bennett BL, Meyers G, Pierce MC. Is the use of physical discipline associated with aggressive behaviors in young children? *Acad Pediatr.* 2017;17(1):34–44

14. Mendez M, Durtschi J, Neppl TK, Stith SM. Corporal punishment and externalizing behaviors in toddlers: the moderating role of positive and harsh parenting. *J Fam Psychol.* 2016;30(8):887–895

15. Lee SJ, Taylor CA, Altschul I, Rice JC. Parental spanking and subsequent risk for child aggression in father-involved families of young children. *Child Youth Serv Rev.* 2013;35(9):1476–1485

16. MacKenzie MJ, Nicklas E, Waldfogel J, Brooks-Gunn J. Corporal punishment and child behavioral and cognitive outcomes through 5 years-of-age: evidence from a contemporary urban birth cohort study. *Infant Child Dev.* 2012;21(1):3–33

17. Taylor CA, Manganello JA, Lee SJ, Rice JC. Mothers' spanking of 3-year-old children and subsequent risk of children's aggressive behavior. *Pediatrics.* 2010;125(5):e1057–e1065

18. Zolotor AJ, Theodore AD, Chang JJ, Berkoff MC, Runyan DK. Speak softly—and forget the stick. Corporal punishment and child physical abuse. *Am J Prev Med.* 2008;35(4):364–369

19. Taylor CA, Hamvas L, Rice J, Newman DL, DeJong W. Perceived social norms, expectations, and attitudes toward corporal punishment among an urban community sample of parents. *J Urban Health.* 2011;88(2):254–269

20. Chung EK, Mathew L, Rothkopf AC, Elo IT, Coyne JC, Culhane JF. Parenting attitudes and infant spanking: the influence of childhood experiences. *Pediatrics.* 2009;124(2):e278–e286

21. American Academy of Pediatrics Committee on Psychosocial Aspects of Child and Family Health. Guidance for effective discipline. *Pediatrics.* 1998;101(4):723–728

22. Hibbard R, Barlow J, MacMillan H; American Academy of Pediatrics Committee on Child Abuse and Neglect; American Academy of Child and Adolescent Psychiatry Child Maltreatment and Violence Committee. Clinical report: psychological maltreatment. *Pediatrics.* 2012;130(2):372–378

23. Friedson M. Authoritarian parenting attitudes and social origin: the multigenerational relationship of socioeconomic position to childrearing values. *Child Abuse Negl.* 2016;51:263–275

24. Rodriguez CM. Parent-child aggression: association with child abuse potential and parenting styles. *Violence Vict.* 2010;25(6):728–741

25. Navarrette R. Spanking isn't child abuse; it's common sense. CNN Web site. http://www.cnn.com/2014/09/18/opinion/navarrette-spanking-kids/index.html. Updated September 18, 2014. Accessed March 1, 2018

26. Mubarak A, Cyr C, St-André M, et al. Child attachment and sensory regulation in psychiatric clinic-referred preschoolers. *Clin Child Psychol Psychiatry.* 2017;22(4):572–587

27. Coppola G, Ponzetti S, Aureli T, Vaughn BE. Patterns of emotion regulation at two years of age: associations with mothers' attachment in a fear eliciting situation. *Attach Hum Dev.* 2016;18(1):16–32

28. Morris AS, Silk JS, Steinberg L, Myers SS, Robinson LR. The role of the family context in the development of emotion regulation. *Soc Dev.* 2007;16(2):361–388

29. Bélanger MÈ, Bernier A, Simard V, Bordeleau S, Carrier J. Viii. Attachment and sleep among toddlers: disentangling attachment security and dependency. *Monogr Soc Res Child Dev.* 2015;80(1):125–140

30. Hardman CA, Christiansen P, Wilkinson LL. Using food to soothe: maternal attachment anxiety is associated with child emotional eating. *Appetite.* 2016;99:91–96

31. Simpson TE, Condon E, Price RM, Finch BK, Sadler LS, Ordway MR. Demystifying infant mental health: what the primary care provider needs to know. *J Pediatr Health Care.* 2016;30(1):38–48

32. Feldman R. Mutual influences between child emotion regulation and parent-child reciprocity support development across the first 10 years of life: implications for developmental psychopathology. *Dev Psychopathol.* 2015;27(4 Pt 1):1007–1023

33. Saunders H, Kraus A, Barone L, Biringen Z. Emotional availability: theory, research, and intervention. *Front Psychol.* 2015;6:1069

34. Murphy TP, Laible DJ, Augustine M, Robeson L. Attachment's links with adolescents' social emotions: the roles of negative emotionality and emotion regulation. *J Genet Psychol.* 2015;176(5):315–329

35. Simard V, Chevalier V, Bédard MM. Sleep and attachment in early childhood: a series of meta-analyses. *Attach Hum Dev.* 2017;19(3):298–321

36. Pennestri MH, Moss E, O'Donnell K, et al. Establishment and consolidation of the sleep-wake cycle as a function of attachment pattern. *Attach Hum Dev.* 2015;17(1):23–42

37. Oosterman M, Schuengel C. Physiological effects of separation and reunion in relation to attachment and temperament in young children. *Dev Psychobiol.* 2007;49(2):119–128

38. Frodi A, Thompson R. Infants' affective responses in the strange situation: effects of prematurity and of quality of attachment. *Child Dev.* 1985;56(5):1280–1290

39. Easterbrooks MA, Lamb ME. The relationship between quality of infant-mother attachment and infant competence in initial encounters with peers. *Child Dev.* 1979; 50(2):380–387

40. Maccoby EE, Feldman SS. Mother-attachment and stranger-reactions in the third year of life. *Monogr Soc Res Child Dev.* 1972;37(1):1–86

41. Kochanska G, Kim S. Early attachment organization with both parents and future behavior problems: from infancy to middle childhood. *Child Dev.* 2013;84(1):283–296

42. Dallaire DH, Weinraub M. Predicting children's separation anxiety at age 6: the contributions of infant-mother attachment security, maternal sensitivity, and maternal separation anxiety. *Attach Hum Dev.* 2005;7(4):393–408

43. Shouldice A, Stevenson-Hinde J. Coping with security distress: the Separation Anxiety Test and attachment classification at 4.5 years. *J Child Psychol Psychiatry.* 1992;33(2):331–348

44. Traub F, Boynton-Jarrett R. Modifiable resilience factors to childhood adversity for clinical pediatric practice. *Pediatrics.* 2017;139(5):e20162569

45. Schilling S, French B, Berkowitz SJ, Dougherty SL, Scribano PV, Wood JN. Child-Adult Relationship Enhancement in Primary Care (PriCARE): a randomized trial of a parent training for child behavior problems. *Acad Pediatr.* 2017;17(1):53–60

46. Kopala-Sibley DC, Dougherty LR, Dyson MW, et al. Early childhood cortisol reactivity moderates the effects of parent-child relationship quality on the development of children's temperament in early childhood. *Dev Sci.* 2017;20(3)

47. Yousafzai AK, Rasheed MA, Rizvi A, Armstrong R, Bhutta ZA. Parenting skills and emotional availability: an RCT. *Pediatrics.* 2015;135(5):e1247–e1257

48. Glascoe FP, Leew S. Parenting behaviors, perceptions, and psychosocial risk: impacts on young children's development. *Pediatrics.* 2010;125(2):313–319

49. Gurwitch RH, Messer EP, Masse J, Olafson E, Boat BW, Putnam FW. Child-Adult Relationship Enhancement (CARE): an evidence-informed program for children with a history of trauma and other behavioral challenges. *Child Abuse Negl.* 2016;53:138–145

50. Bjørseth Å, Wichstrøm L. Effectiveness of parent-child interaction therapy (PCIT) in the treatment of young children's behavior problems. A randomized controlled study. *PLoS One.* 2016;11(9):e0159845

51. Niec LN, Barnett ML, Prewett MS, Shanley Chatham JR. Group parent-child interaction therapy: a randomized control trial for the treatment of conduct problems in young children. *J Consult Clin Psychol.* 2016;84(8):682–698

52. Thomas R, Herschell AD. Parent-child interaction therapy: a manualized intervention for the therapeutic child welfare sector. *Child Abuse Negl.* 2013;37(8):578–584

53. Thomas R, Zimmer-Gembeck MJ. Behavioral outcomes of parent-child interaction therapy and Triple P-Positive Parenting Program: a review and meta-analysis. *J Abnorm Child Psychol.* 2007;35(3):475–495

54. Guild DJ, Toth SL, Handley ED, Rogosch FA, Cicchetti D. Attachment security mediates the longitudinal association between child-parent psychotherapy and peer relations for toddlers of depressed mothers. *Dev Psychopathol.* 2017;29(2):587–600

55. Stronach EP, Toth SL, Rogosch F, Cicchetti D. Preventive interventions and sustained attachment security in maltreated children. *Dev Psychopathol.* 2013;25(4 Pt 1):919–930

56. Lieberman AF, Ghosh Ippen C, Van Horn P. Child-parent psychotherapy: 6-month follow-up of a randomized controlled trial. *J Am Acad Child Adolesc Psychiatry.* 2006;45(8):913–918

57. Lind T, Lee Raby K, Caron EB, Roben CK, Dozier M. Enhancing executive functioning among toddlers in foster care with an attachment-based intervention. *Dev Psychopathol.* 2017;29(2):575–586

58. Yarger HA, Hoye JR, Dozier M. Trajectories of change in Attachment and Biobehavioral Catch-up among high-risk mothers: a randomized clinical trial. *Infant Ment Health J.* 2016;37(5):525–536

59. Bernard K, Hostinar CE, Dozier M. Intervention effects on diurnal cortisol rhythms of child protective services-referred infants in early childhood: preschool follow-up results of a randomized clinical trial. *JAMA Pediatr.* 2015;169(2):112–119

60. Bernard K, Dozier M, Bick J, Lewis-Morrarty E, Lindhiem O, Carlson E. Enhancing attachment organization among maltreated children: results of a randomized clinical trial. *Child Dev.* 2012;83(2):623–636

61. Sinha R. Role of addiction and stress neurobiology on food intake and obesity. *Biol Psychol.* 2018;131:5–13

62. Cardel MI, Johnson SL, Beck J, et al. The effects of experimentally manipulated social status on acute eating behavior: a randomized, crossover pilot study. *Physiol Behav.* 2016;162:93–101

63. Hardy LL, Reinten-Reynolds T, Espinel P, Zask A, Okely AD. Prevalence and correlates of low fundamental movement skill competency in children. *Pediatrics.* 2012;130(2):e390–e398

64. Logan SW, Robinson LE, Wilson AE, Lucas WA. Getting the fundamentals of movement: a meta-analysis of the effectiveness of motor skill interventions in children. *Child Care Health Dev.* 2012;38(3):305–315

65. Kushner RF, Sarwer DB. Medical and behavioral evaluation of patients with obesity. *Psychiatr Clin North Am.* 2011;34(4):797–812

66. Cliff DP, Okely AD, Magarey AM. Movement skill mastery in a clinical sample of overweight and obese children. *Int J Pediatr Obes.* 2011;6(5-6):473–475

67. Wells NM, Evans GW, Beavis A, Ong AD. Early childhood poverty, cumulative risk exposure, and body mass index trajectories through young adulthood. *Am J Public Health.* 2010;100(12):2507–2512

68. Janicke DM, Harman JS, Kelleher KJ, Zhang J. The association of psychiatric diagnoses, health service use, and expenditures in children with obesity-related health conditions. *J Pediatr Psychol.* 2009;34(1):79–88

69. Machado TD, Dalle Molle R, Reis RS, et al. Interaction between perceived maternal care, anxiety symptoms, and the neurobehavioral response to palatable foods in adolescents. *Stress.* 2016;19(3):287–294

70. Evans GW, Jones-Rounds ML, Belojevic G, Vermeylen F. Family income and childhood obesity in eight European cities: the mediating roles of neighborhood characteristics and physical activity. *Soc Sci Med.* 2012;75(3):477–481

71. Evans GW, Fuller-Rowell TE, Doan SN. Childhood cumulative risk and obesity: the mediating role of self-regulatory ability. *Pediatrics.* 2012;129(1):e68–e73

72. Suglia SF, Duarte CS, Chambers EC, Boynton-Jarrett R. Social and behavioral risk factors for obesity in early childhood. *J Dev Behav Pediatr.* 2013;34(8):549–556

73. Ryan-Ibarra S, Sanchez-Vaznaugh EV, Leung C, Induni M. The relationship between food insecurity and overweight/obesity differs by birthplace and length of US residence. *Public Health Nutr.* 2017;20(4):671–677

74. Dhurandhar EJ. The food-insecurity obesity paradox: a resource scarcity hypothesis. *Physiol Behav.* 2016;162:88–92

75. Speirs KE, Fiese BH; STRONG Kids Research Team. The relationship between food insecurity and BMI for preschool children. *Matern Child Health J.* 2016;20(4):925–933

76. Kaur J, Lamb MM, Ogden CL. The association between food insecurity and obesity in children—the National Health and Nutrition Examination Survey. *J Acad Nutr Diet.* 2015;115(5):751–758

77. Gross RS, Mendelsohn AL, Fierman AH, Racine AD, Messito MJ. Food insecurity and obesogenic maternal infant feeding styles and practices in low-income families. *Pediatrics.* 2012;130(2):254–261

78. Shah R, Sobotka SA, Chen YF, Msall ME. Positive parenting practices, health disparities, and developmental progress. *Pediatrics.* 2015;136(2):318–326

79. Bacchini D, Licenziati MR, Affuso G, et al. The interplay among BMI z-score, peer victmization, and self-concept in outpatient children and adolescents with overweight or obesity. *Child Obes.* 2017;13(3):242–249

80. Odar Stough C, Merianos A, Nabors L, Peugh J. Prevalence and predictors of bullying behavior among overweight and obese youth in a nationally representative sample. *Child Obes.* 2016;12(4):263–271

81. Puhl RM, Latner JD, O'Brien K, Luedicke J, Forhan M, Danielsdottir S. Cross-national perspectives about weight-based bullying in youth: nature, extent and remedies. *Pediatr Obes.* 2016;11(4):241–250

82. Jansen PW, Verlinden M, Dommisse-van Berkel A, et al. Teacher and peer reports of overweight and bullying among young primary school children. *Pediatrics.* 2014;134(3):473–480

83. Garg A, Boynton-Jarrett R, Dworkin PH. Avoiding the unintended consequences of screening for social determinants of health. *JAMA.* 2016;316(8):813–814

84. Beach SR, Lei MK, Brody GH, et al. Parenting, socioeconomic status risk, and later young adult health: exploration of opposing indirect effects via DNA methylation. *Child Dev.* 2016;87(1):111–121

85. Lam LL, Emberly E, Fraser HB, et al. Factors underlying variable DNA methylation in a human community cohort. *Proc Natl Acad Sci U S A.* 2012;109(Suppl 2):17253–17260

86. Luby J, Belden A, Botteron K, et al. The effects of poverty on childhood brain development: the mediating effect of caregiving and stressful life events. *JAMA Pediatr.* 2013;167(12):1135–1142

87. Kim P, Evans GW, Angstadt M, et al. Effects of childhood poverty and chronic stress on emotion regulatory brain function in adulthood. *Proc Natl Acad Sci U S A.* 2013;110(46):18442–18447

88. Granström F, Eriksson HG, Molarius A. Economic stress and condescending treatment in childhood and adult self-rated health: results from a population study in Sweden. *BMC Public Health.* 2017;17(1):489

89. Giovanelli A, Reynolds AJ, Mondi CF, Ou SR. Adverse childhood experiences and adult well-being in a low-income, urban cohort. *Pediatrics.* 2016;137(4):e20154016

90. Non AL, Román JC, Gross CL, et al. Early childhood social disadvantage is associated with poor health behaviours in adulthood. *Ann Hum Biol.* 2016;43(2):144–153

91. Wade R Jr, Cronholm PF, Fein JA, et al. Household and community-level Adverse Childhood Experiences and adult health outcomes in a diverse urban population. *Child Abuse Negl.* 2016;52:135–145

92. Non AL, Rewak M, Kawachi I, et al. Childhood social disadvantage, cardiometabolic risk, and chronic disease in adulthood. *Am J Epidemiol.* 2014;180(3):263–271

93. Johnson SL, Wibbels E, Wilkinson R. Economic inequality is related to cross-national prevalence of psychotic symptoms. *Soc Psychiatry Psychiatr Epidemiol.* 2015;50(12):1799–1807

94. Pickett KE, Wilkinson RG. The ethical and policy implications of research on income inequality and child well-being. *Pediatrics.* 2015;135(Suppl 2):S39–S47

95. Nowatzki NR. Wealth inequality and health: a political economy perspective. *Int J Health Serv.* 2012;42(3):403–424

96. Biggs B, King L, Basu S, Stuckler D. Is wealthier always healthier? The impact of national income level, inequality, and poverty on public health in Latin America. *Soc Sci Med.* 2010;71(2):266–273

97. American Academy of Pediatrics Council on Community Pediatrics. Poverty and child health in the United States. *Pediatrics.* 2016;137(4):e20160339

98. Douglass F. BrainyQuote Web site. https://www.brainyquote.com/quotes/frederick_douglass_201574. Accessed March 1, 2018

99. Ohio Chapter of the American Academy of Pediatrics. Building "Piece" of Mind handouts. http://ohioaap.org/projects/building-mental-wellness/building-piece-of-mind-handouts. Accessed March 1, 2018

100. National Scientific Counsel on the Developing Child. *Young Children Develop in an Environment of Relationships: Working Paper No. 1.* 2004. http://developingchild.harvard. edu/resources/wp1. Accessed March 1, 2018

101. Thompson JL, Sebire SJ, Kesten JM, et al. How parents perceive screen viewing in their 5-6 year old child within the context of their own screen viewing time: a mixed-methods study. *BMC Public Health.* 2017;17(1):471

102. Zuckerman B, Augustyn M. Books and reading: evidence-based standard of care whose time has come. *Acad Pediatr.* 2011;11(1):11–17

103. Zuckerman B, Khandekar A. Reach Out and Read: evidence based approach to promoting early child development. *Curr Opin Pediatr.* 2010;22(4):539–544

104. Walker SP, Chang SM, Vera-Hernández M, Grantham-McGregor S. Early childhood stimulation benefits adult competence and reduces violent behavior. *Pediatrics.* 2011;127(5):849–857

105. Dodds M, Nicholson L, Muse B, Osborn LM. Group health supervision visits more effective than individual visits in delivering health care information. *Pediatrics.* 1993;91(3):668–670

106. Rushton FE, Byrne WW, Darden PM, McLeigh J. Enhancing child safety and well-being through pediatric group well-child care and home visitation: the Well Baby Plus Program. *Child Abuse Negl.* 2015;41:182–189

107. Machuca H, Arevalo S, Hackley B, et al. Well baby group care: evaluation of a promising intervention for primary obesity prevention in toddlers. *Child Obes.* 2016;12(3):171–178

108. Bauer NS, Szczepaniak D, Sullivan PD, et al. Group visits to improve pediatric attention-deficit hyperactivity disorder chronic care management. *J Dev Behav Pediatr.* 2015;36(8): 553–561

109. Minkovitz CS, Strobino D, Mistry KB, et al. Healthy Steps for Young Children: sustained results at 5.5 years. *Pediatrics.* 2007;120(3):e658–e668

110. Johnston BD, Huebner CE, Anderson ML, Tyll LT, Thompson RS. Healthy steps in an integrated delivery system: child and parent outcomes at 30 months. *Arch Pediatr Adolesc Med.* 2006;160(8):793–800

111. Zuckerman B, Parker S, Kaplan-Sanoff M, Augustyn M, Barth MC. Healthy Steps: a case study of innovation in pediatric practice. *Pediatrics.* 2004;114(3):820–826

112. Weisleder A, Cates CB, Dreyer BP, et al. Promotion of positive parenting and prevention of socioemotional disparities. *Pediatrics.* 2016;137(2):e20153239

113. Mendelsohn AL, Huberman HS, Berkule SB, Brockmeyer CA, Morrow LM, Dreyer BP. Primary care strategies for promoting parent-child interactions and school readiness in at-risk families: the Bellevue Project for Early Language, Literacy, and Education Success. *Arch Pediatr Adolesc Med.* 2011;165(1):33–41

114. Mendelsohn AL, Valdez PT, Flynn V, et al. Use of videotaped interactions during pediatric well-child care: impact at 33 months on parenting and on child development. *J Dev Behav Pediatr.* 2007;28(3):206–212

115. Institute for Healthcare Improvement. The Triple Aim. Optimizing health, care and cost. *Healthc Exec.* 2009;24(1):64–66

116. Berwick DM, Nolan TW, Whittington J. The triple aim: care, health, and cost. *Health Aff (Millwood).* 2008;27(3):759–769

117. Bodenheimer T, Sinsky C. From triple to quadruple aim: care of the patient requires care of the provider. *Ann Fam Med.* 2014;12(6):573–576

118. Felitti VJ, Anda RF, Nordenberg D, et al. Relationship of childhood abuse and household dysfunction to many of the leading causes of death in adults. The Adverse Childhood Experiences (ACE) Study. *Am J Prev Med.* 1998;14(4):245–258

119. Stein RE, Storfer-Isser A, Kerker BD, et al. Does length of developmental behavioral pediatrics training matter? *Acad Pediatr.* 2017;17(1):61–67

120. Stein REK. Are we on the right track? Examining the role of developmental behavioral pediatrics. *Pediatrics.* 2015;135(4):589–591

121. Horwitz SM, Caspary G, Storfer-Isser A, et al. Is developmental and behavioral pediatrics training related to perceived responsibility for treating mental health problems? *Acad Pediatr.* 2010;10(4):252–259

122. Garner AS, Storfer-Isser A, Szilagyi M, et al. Promoting early brain and child development: perceived barriers and the utilization of resources to address them. *Acad Pediatr.* 2017;17(7):697–705

123. Szilagyi M, Kerker BD, Storfer-Isser A, et al. Factors associated with whether pediatricians inquire about parents' adverse childhood experiences. *Acad Pediatr.* 2016;16(7):668–675

124. Center on the Developing Child at Harvard University. *Supportive Relationships and Active Skill-Building Strengthen the Foundations of Resilience: Working Paper No. 13.* 2015. https://developingchild.harvard.edu/resources/supportive-relationships-and-active-skill-building-strengthen-the-foundations-of-resilience. Accessed March 1, 2018

125. National Scientific Counsel on the Developing Child. *The Timing and Quality of Early Experiences Combine to Shape Brain Architecture: Working Paper No. 5.* 2007. https://developingchild.harvard.edu/resources/the-timing-and-quality-of-early-experiences-combine-to-shape-brain-architecture. Accessed March 1, 2018

126. Zuckerman B. Two-generation pediatric care: a modest proposal. *Pediatrics.* 2016;137(1):e20153447

127. Kuo AA, Etzel RA, Chilton LA, Watson C, Gorski PA. Primary care pediatrics and public health: meeting the needs of today's children. *Am J Public Health.* 2012;102(12):e17–e23

128. Goldhagen J. Integrating pediatrics and public health. *Pediatrics.* 2005;115(Suppl 3):1202–1208

Chapter 10

Implications for Pediatric Advocacy and Public Policy

● ●

When you can't make them see the light,
make them feel the heat.

– *Ronald Reagan[1]*

● ●

The ecobiodevelopmental (EBD) model forces pediatricians to think developmentally, to go upstream, and to acknowledge that adverse childhood experiences (ACEs), toxic stress, and relational health have pivotal roles in determining developmental outcomes and life course trajectories. In the previous chapter, we discussed the implications of the EBD model for the family-centered pediatric medical home (FCPMH), and we presented a few initial steps toward the translation of developmental science into pediatric practice. In this chapter, we will discuss the implications of thinking developmentally for pediatric advocacy, and we will present a few initial objectives for the translation of developmental science into public policy.

Principles of Pediatric Advocacy

As pediatric clinicians who think developmentally, our advocacy includes the following essential elements:

1. **We advocate for all children, regardless of their place, race, or ACE.** The mission of the American Academy of Pediatrics (AAP) has been "to attain optimal physical, mental, and social health and well-being for all infants, children, adolescents, and young adults."[2] The EBD model suggests that to attain optimal outcomes for all children, we need to work

tirelessly to improve the ecology in which they develop, regardless of the zip code where they live, their family's heritage, or the adversities they may have encountered in the past.

2. **Our advocacy is grounded in the biology of development.** Although the ethical and economic arguments to support young families and their children are persuasive, pediatric advocacy is grounded in the fact that many so-called adult-onset diseases are actually adult-*manifest* conditions with their origins in childhood.[3] Recent advances in epigenetics and developmental neurosciences explain how the early childhood ecology is biologically embedded, influencing developmental outcomes across the life span.[4,5] The mind may not recall pivotal experiences in early childhood, but the body remembers and continues to react accordingly.

3. **We use a developmentally informed model of disease and wellness because both are the result of an ongoing but cumulative dance between ecology and biology.** The child's experiences and relationships interact with the child's genome and brain to drive development in childhood and beyond.[3] The EBD model explains why investments in early childhood ecology are necessary to improve developmental outcomes and optimize life course trajectories.

4. **We recognize that children have deficiency needs (ie, physiologic, safety, connection, and esteem) that must be met for children to develop in a healthy manner.** When these deficiency needs are not adequately met, toxic stress responses alter the child's genome and brain, making self-actualization and the fulfillment of the child's biological potential more difficult to achieve.

5. **Our advocacy highlights the fact that safe, stable, and nurturing relationships are the antidote to childhood toxic stress.** Safe, stable, and nurturing relationships allow children's deficiency needs to be met, releasing the brake on their early brain and child development. Parents and caregivers who place a premium on the relational health of the dyad buffer their children's toxic stress responses, allow their children to learn pivotal social and emotional skills, and prepare their children to respond to future adversity in a healthy, adaptive manner.

6. **We are compelled to recognize and address prominent barriers to relational health.** Unmet adult deficiency needs (ie, physiologic, safety, connection, and esteem) and the so-called social determinants of health can make it harder for parents, other caregivers, and communities as a whole to provide the safe, stable, and nurturing relationships needed to meet a child's deficiency needs. A 2-generation approach is, therefore, necessary—help parents and caregivers to help their children.[6]

7. **We reaffirm the therapeutic relationship between the pediatric health care professional and the child's family and caregivers as the foundation for all that we do.** Potential barriers to therapeutic relationships, like health care provider time constraints, limits to the continuity of care, and an increasing emphasis on documentation and billing concerns over the actual provision of care (eg, electronic medical record use, meaningful use requirements), threaten the quality of care provided, the family's satisfaction with the care, and the health care provider's professional satisfaction.

8. **We recognize that complex, intractable problems like childhood adversity, poverty, and violence require a public health approach.** With a public health approach, programs are not isolated but integrated vertically and horizontally into a collaborative system of care. Vertical integration is necessary because children, families, and communities differ in their relative strengths and weaknesses, so successful systems will include varying levels of care (eg, universal preventions, targeted interventions, indicated treatments) and will match those levels of care with the particular area of greatest need. Horizontal integration across the medical, educational, and social sectors is necessary because even the best health care system in the world cannot compensate for deficits in educational and social services. Similarly, the education system cannot compensate for inaccessible medical or social services.

9. **We advocate for a public health approach that not only prevents, mitigates, and treats toxic stress but actively promotes, eliminates barriers to, and repairs relational health.** The FCPMH is well positioned to advocate for and participate in local systems of care that adopt this broad public health approach to toxic stress and relational health. But the FCPMH is not likely to accomplish all these noble objectives in isolation. To promote wellness and improve life course trajectories, a coordinated, cross-sector, and collaborative approach is needed to improve the lives of young children, their families, and their communities. Consequently, 2 essential elements of pediatric advocacy are the clarification of general goals that cut across sectors and the provision of specific policy recommendations that must be heeded to meet those general goals.

General Goals and Specific Policy Recommendations

Prior to the 2016 US presidential election, the AAP published *Blueprint for Children: How the Next President Can Build a Foundation for a Healthy Future.*[7] In this document, the AAP outlined general goals and specific policy recommendations for healthy children, secure families, and strong communities. An abridged and amended version of this document appears in Appendix B. Here we highlight a few of these general goals and specific policy recommendations for *building healthy, resilient children* through *strong families* and *communities that care.* This reflects the public health approach advocated throughout this book.

Building Healthy, Resilient Children

GENERAL GOALS

To build healthy, resilient children, all children will have their essential, biological needs met (ie, physiologic, safety, connection, and self-esteem). Regardless of their immigration status, all children will have access to affordable health care coverage that is comprehensive and recognizes the benefits of 2-generational care. Ideally, all children will receive their primary care in a medical home that is family centered, and they will have access to any needed subspecialty and mental health care services.

SPECIFIC POLICY RECOMMENDATIONS

Specific policy recommendations to build healthy, resilient children include ensuring that all public and private health plans include essential health benefit packages that are comprehensive, well defined, and appropriate for pediatric care and include 2-generational benefits.[8] Such packages must include a broad range of services, including evidence-based programs that promote relational health (eg, Reach Out and Read,[9,10] home visiting programs[11-13]), eliminate barriers to relational health (eg, Health Leads[14]; Well-child Care Visit, Evaluation, Community Resources, Advocacy, Referral, Education [WE CARE][15,16]; iScreen[17,18]; medicolegal partnerships[19]), and repair relational health (eg, child-parent psychotherapy,[20] parent-child interaction therapy[21]). Children will also benefit from improved and innovative financing packages that incentivize high-quality, team-based care in FCPMHs that incorporate Bright Futures guidelines[22] and Early and Periodic Screening, Diagnosis, and Treatment services. To support disadvantaged children, access to Medicaid services must be not only maintained but improved by simplifying eligibility processes, reducing bureaucratic barriers to care, and streamlining enrollment; support for the Children's Health Insurance Program must be maintained; and loan repayment programs and other incentives must be extended to pediatricians and subspecialists who work in underserved areas or care for low-income families. Finally, to build healthy, resilient children, confidentiality rules must be revised to promote collaboration among the medical home, the educational community, and social services and to ensure that children's essential biological needs are being met.

Building Strong Families

GENERAL GOALS

To build strong families, more must be done to support families as they nurture within their children the behaviors and skills necessary for healthy and productive life course trajectories. General goals to support strong families will include all the goals outlined previously for building healthy, resilient children, because today's children will parent the next generation of families. In addition, all families will have access to work that provides a stable and adequate income and family-friendly benefits; safe, secure housing; adequate, healthy, and nutritious food throughout the year; and affordable, safe, and high-quality child care. Most importantly, all families will have access to community resources that support relational health and the adoption of positive parenting practices.

SPECIFIC POLICY RECOMMENDATIONS

Specific policy recommendations to build strong families must include opportunities to lift young families out of poverty. Raising the minimum wage, offering job training, strengthening the earned income tax credit and child tax credit, expanding the Temporary Assistance for Needy Families program, strengthening the Supplemental Nutrition Assistance Program, and enhancing family and medical leave[23] are all opportunities to support families and promote relational mode over survival mode. To make affordable and high-quality child care accessible for all families, resources must be directed toward the Office of Child Care in the Administration for Children and Families, and the Child Care and Development Block Grant Act must be expanded and strengthened. To improve access to affordable and safe housing, federal rental assistance must be expanded. To ensure access to adequate nutrition, federal programs like the Special Supplemental Nutrition Program for Women, Infants, and Children; the National School Lunch Program and School Breakfast Program; and the Summer Food Service Program must be strengthened and expanded. Finally, programs for at-risk parents, like the Maternal, Infant, and Early Childhood Home Visiting Program, must be expanded to identify and connect parents with community services that treat depression or substance abuse, mitigate other precipitants of toxic stress, and promote child well-being. To build strong families, peer and community social supports must be enhanced through programs like Centering Pregnancy,[24] Centering Parenting,[25,26] and Legacy for Children.[27]

Building Communities That Care

GENERAL GOALS

Because it is far easier to build healthy, resilient children and strong, secure families when they live in communities that care, more must be done to support relational health at the community level. General goals toward building communities that care will include all the general goals outlined previously for building strong families, because families make communities. Much like individuals, it may be hard for families to think relationally when they are in survival mode. When families are safe and secure in communities where they feel accepted, they may be more likely to engage in how their community nurtures and cares for other families (eg, voting, advocating, simply setting the tone). Hence, as general goals, all communities will work collaboratively to keep their neighborhoods safe from violence and free of environmental hazards (eg, lead); provide high-quality early education programs; support public health systems that protect children from infectious diseases and promote maternal and child health; promote relational health by denouncing racism, hatred, and oppression; and proactively support the disadvantaged within their midst.

SPECIFIC POLICY RECOMMENDATIONS

Specific policy recommendations to build communities that care include more federally funded research to build the evidence base for a public health response to violence in all its varied forms (ie, physical, psychological, racial, and economic). To keep communities safe, efforts must be made to ensure that firearms do not get into the wrong hands by passing comprehensive, commonsense gun violence prevention measures (eg, banning assault weapons, improving background checks). In addition, our aging and outdated infrastructure must be addressed to reduce exposures to lead and increase disaster preparedness. To promote inclusion and minimize disparities, efforts must be made to increase the number of children in prekindergarten education and proven, high-quality early learning programs, such as Head Start and Early Head Start; provide low-income neighborhoods with resources to ensure that all children and adolescents have access to safe and desirable opportunities for play and active lifestyles; implement formalized social and emotional learning in schools[28,29]; and expand evidence-based programs that promote restorative justice.[30–32]

Although the EBD model supports all these goals and policy recommendations as opportunities to improve childhood ecologies and developmental outcomes, this list is by no means complete. Recall that the EBD model is grounded squarely in the unifying developmental science that underlies not only health outcomes but educational success, civic engagement, and economic productivity. Thinking developmentally begins to break down the barriers between traditional policy silos and informs not only health policy but educational policy, social policy, and even economic policy.

Moving Forward by Generating Political Will

Dr Julius Richmond, the cofounder of Head Start, former Surgeon General of the United States, and an exemplar advocate for children, once published a schema for successful advocacy that included 3 key domains: the *knowledge base,* a *social strategy,* and the *political will.*[33,34]

Knowledge Base: The Why

In Dr Richmond's model, the knowledge base refers to the *why.* The advances in developmental science discussed in Part 1 explain

- Why the early childhood ecology is so instrumental: it sets the stage for disease and health decades later.
- Why unmet needs make self-actualization more difficult: they make it harder for young children to fulfill their biological potential and for parents to be the best possible versions of themselves.
- Why safe, stable, and nurturing relationships are the antidote to childhood adversity and toxic stress, and why relational health is the foundation for building healthy and resilient children, strong families, and communities that care.
- Why investments in the early childhood ecology are necessary to improve developmental outcomes, not only in heath but in educational success and economic productivity.

The EBD model may serve as a simple, approachable tool for educating parents, policy makers, and a wide array of professionals about the way *nurture* (experiences with the ecology) and *nature* (the genome) interact in a dynamic but cumulative manner to drive development not only in childhood but across the life span. One of the overarching goals of this book is to explain the knowledge base that is emerging from advances in epigenetics, neurosciences, and life course sciences.

Social Strategy: The How

In Dr Richmond's model, a social strategy refers to the *how:* How do we get from where we currently are to where we want to be? How is the knowledge base to be applied? How will we know if the knowledge base is being applied successfully? How will we define and measure the discrete steps toward our ultimate goal? As Dr Richmond liked to say, "You cannot get very far if you do not know where you are going."[34]

The implications of thinking developmentally discussed in Part 2 provide an initial road map for how to translate the knowledge base into practice and policy. Regardless of whether the EBD model is being applied to children, families, communities, or pediatric practice, we have argued for a public health approach that prevents, mitigates, and treats toxic stress while also promoting, eliminating barriers to, and repairing relational health. To have an effect, discrete programs will need to be integrated vertically and horizontally into the local system of care. The potential policy objectives mentioned in this chapter are initial steps in the journey toward building healthy children, strong families, and communities that care, but many other steps are likely to be needed as well. For example, a mass media campaign (as has been done with the risks of tobacco[35] or the use of seat belts[36,37]) will likely be needed to increase awareness and generate the political will to invest in relational health.

Political Will: The Who

In Dr Richmond's model, the political will refers to the *who:* Who needs to understand the knowledge base and buy into the social strategy to get the job done? One of the challenges to pediatric advocacy is that children do not vote and they have not (yet!) formed a political action committee to get the political attention they deserve. But pediatricians vote, as do teachers, social workers, child care professionals, judges, and forward-thinking economists. Most importantly, parents also vote, but they may not recognize how public policy affects a child's ecology, biology, and developmental potential. They may not understand how relational health releases the brake on a child's biological potential, allowing the child's talents to benefit us all. But if parents, grandparents, and all professionals who care for children voted for kids first and foremost, the political pressure for legislators to also *put kids first* would be tremendous. As Ronald Reagan once said, "When you can't make them see the light, make them feel the heat."[1] Despite the strong emotions underlying divisive politics, pediatricians grounded in the EBD model will steadfastly advocate for programs and policies that support relational health because it is only through communities that care that families will be strong and children will be healthy and resilient.

References

1. Reagan R. BrainyQuote Web site. https://www.brainyquote.com/quotes/ronald_reagan_383264. Accessed March 1, 2018
2. American Academy of Pediatrics. AAP facts. https://www.aap.org/en-us/about-the-aap/aap-facts/pages/aap-facts.aspx. Accessed March 1, 2018

3. Garner AS. Thinking developmentally: the next evolution in models of health. *J Dev Behav Pediatr.* 2016;37(7):579–584

4. Shonkoff JP, Garner AS; American Academy of Pediatrics Committee on Psychosocial Aspects of Child and Family Health; Committee on Early Childhood, Adoption, and Dependent Care; Section on Developmental and Behavioral Pediatrics. Technical report: the lifelong effects of early childhood adversity and toxic stress. *Pediatrics.* 2012;129(1):e232–e246

5. American Academy of Pediatrics Committee on Psychosocial Aspects of Child and Family Health; Committee on Early Childhood, Adoption, and Dependent Care; Section on Developmental and Behavioral Pediatrics. Policy statement: early childhood adversity, toxic stress, and the role of the pediatrician: translating developmental science into lifelong health. *Pediatrics.* 2012;129(1):e224–e231

6. Center on the Developing Child at Harvard University. *Supportive Relationships and Active Skill-Building Strengthen the Foundations of Resilience: Working Paper No. 13.* 2015. https://developingchild.harvard.edu/resources/supportive-relationships-and-active-skill-building-strengthen-the-foundations-of-resilience. Accessed March 1, 2018

7. American Academy of Pediatrics. *Blueprint for Children: How the Next President Can Build a Foundation for a Healthy Future.* https://www.aap.org/en-us/Documents/BluePrintForChildren.pdf. Published September 2016. Accessed March 1, 2018

8. Davis MM. Evidence for a uniform Medicaid eligibility threshold for children and parents. *Pediatrics.* 2017;140(6):e20173236

9. Zuckerman B, Augustyn M. Books and reading: evidence-based standard of care whose time has come. *Acad Pediatr.* 2011;11(1):11–17

10. Zuckerman B, Khandekar A. Reach Out and Read: evidence based approach to promoting early child development. *Curr Opin Pediatr.* 2010;22(4):539–544

11. Garner AS. Home visiting and the biology of toxic stress: opportunities to address early childhood adversity. *Pediatrics.* 2013;132(Suppl 2):S65–S73

12. Toomey SL, Cheng TL; APA-AAP Workgroup on the Family-Centered Medical Home. Home visiting and the family-centered medical home: synergistic services to promote child health. *Acad Pediatr.* 2013;13(1):3–5

13. Moss E, Dubois-Comtois K, Cyr C, Tarabulsy GM, St-Laurent D, Bernier A. Efficacy of a home-visiting intervention aimed at improving maternal sensitivity, child attachment, and behavioral outcomes for maltreated children: a randomized control trial. *Dev Psychopathol.* 2011;23(1):195–210

14. HealthLeads. Our vision. https://healthleadsusa.org/about-us/vision. Accessed March 1, 2018

15. Garg A, Toy S, Tripodis Y, Silverstein M, Freeman E. Addressing social determinants of health at well child care visits: a cluster RCT. *Pediatrics.* 2015;135(2):e296–e304

16. Garg A, Butz AM, Dworkin PH, Lewis RA, Thompson RE, Serwint JR. Improving the management of family psychosocial problems at low-income children's well-child care visits: the WE CARE Project. *Pediatrics.* 2007;120(3):547–558

17. Gottlieb LM, Hessler D, Long D, et al. Effects of social needs screening and in-person service navigation on child health: a randomized clinical trial. *JAMA Pediatr.* 2016;170(11):e162521

18. Gottlieb L, Hessler D, Long D, Amaya A, Adler N. A randomized trial on screening for social determinants of health: the iScreen study. *Pediatrics.* 2014;134(6):e1611–e1618

19. Sege R, Preer G, Morton SJ, et al. Medical-legal strategies to improve infant health care: a randomized trial. *Pediatrics.* 2015;136(1):97–106

20. Guild DJ, Toth SL, Handley ED, Rogosch FA, Cicchetti D. Attachment security mediates the longitudinal association between child-parent psychotherapy and peer relations for toddlers of depressed mothers. *Dev Psychopathol.* 2017;29(2):587–600

21. Bjørseth Å, Wichstrøm L. Effectiveness of parent-child interaction therapy (PCIT) in the treatment of young children's behavior problems. A randomized controlled study. *PLoS One.* 2016;11(9):e0159845

22. Hagan JF, Shaw JS, Duncan PM, eds. *Bright Futures: Guidelines for Health Supervision of Infants, Children, and Adolescents.* 4th ed. Elk Grove Village, IL: American Academy of Pediatrics; 2017

23. American Academy of Pediatrics Council on Community Pediatrics. Poverty and child health in the United States. *Pediatrics.* 2016;137(4):e20160339

24. Felder JN, Epel E, Lewis JB, et al. Depressive symptoms and gestational length among pregnant adolescents: cluster randomized control trial of CenteringPregnancy plus group prenatal care. *J Consult Clin Psychol.* 2017;85(6):574–584

25. Bloomfield J, Rising SS. CenteringParenting: an innovative dyad model for group mother-infant care. *J Midwifery Womens Health.* 2013;58(6):683–689

26. Mittal P. Centering parenting: pilot implementation of a group model for teaching family medicine residents well-child care. *Perm J.* 2011;15(4):40–41

27. Perou R, Elliott MN, Visser SN, et al. Legacy for Children: a pair of randomized controlled trials of a public health model to improve developmental outcomes among children in poverty. *BMC Public Health.* 2012;12:691

28. Durlak JA, Weissberg RP, Dymnicki AB, Taylor RD, Schellinger KB. The impact of enhancing students' social and emotional learning: a meta-analysis of school-based universal interventions. *Child Dev.* 2011;82(1):405–432

29. Payton J, Weissberg RP, Durlak JA, et al. *The Positive Impact of Social and Emotional Learning for Kindergarten to Eighth-Grade Students: Findings From Three Scientific Reviews.* https://www.casel.org/wp-content/uploads/2016/06/the-positive-impact-of-social-and-emotional-learning-for-kindergarten-to-eighth-grade-students-executive-summary.pdf. Published December 2008. Accessed March 1, 2018

30. Armour M, Sliva S. How does it work? Mechanisms of action in an in-prison restorative justice program. *Int J Offender Ther Comp Criminol.* 2018;62(3):759–784

31. Riedl K, Jensen K, Call J, Tomasello M. Restorative justice in children. *Curr Biol.* 2015;25(13):1731–1735

32. Koss MP. The RESTORE program of restorative justice for sex crimes: vision, process, and outcomes. *J Interpers Violence.* 2014;29(9):1623–1660

33. Richmond JB, Kotelchuck M. The effects of political process on the delivery of health services. In: McGuire CFR, Gorr D, Richard R, eds. *Handbook of Health Professions Education.* San Francisco, CA: Jossey-Bass; 1983:386

34. Palfrey JS. *Child Health in America: Making a Difference through Advocacy.* Baltimore, MD: Johns Hopkins University Press; 2006

35. Cummings KM, Proctor RN. The changing public image of smoking in the United States: 1964-2014. *Cancer Epidemiol Biomarkers Prev.* 2014;23(1):32–36

36. Debinski B, Clegg Smith K, Gielen A. Public opinion on motor vehicle-related injury prevention policies: a systematic review of a decade of research. *Traffic Inj Prev.* 2014;15(3):243–251

37. Vasudevan V, Nambisan SS, Singh AK, Pearl T. Effectiveness of media and enforcement campaigns in increasing seat belt usage rates in a state with a secondary seat belt law. *Traffic Inj Prev.* 2009;10(4):330–339

Epilogue

Hopes and Dreams

* *

Every child must be made aware
Every child must be made to care
Care enough for his fellow man
To give all the love that he can
I pray my wish will come true
For my child and your child too

– "Peace on Earth/Little Drummer Boy"[1]

* *

When asked if writing was a chore, American sportswriter Walter
Wellesley "Red" Smith wryly replied, "Why, no. You simply sit down
at the typewriter, open your veins, and bleed."[2] Similarly, the subtitle for a
popular guidebook on the craft of writing is *Embodying Your Authentic Voice.*[3]
For any writing to be authentic and persuasive, it must be born from a voice, a
vision, or a kernel of truth that is deeply held and very personal. Because our
intention from the very beginning was to produce a book that was squarely
grounded in the latest advances in developmental science, we have tried to
avoid language that might be perceived as overtly biased, subjective, specu-
lative, or partisan. But this book has also been born out of our passion to
provide better care for young children and their families, to improve a health
system that is broken and unsustainable, and to challenge social norms that
either ignore or actively propagate the widening disparities and inequities that
are eroding our collective relational health. So, if we haven't already tipped our
hand, let us be clear about what our hopes and dreams are for this book.

Our Hopes: "Every Child Must Be Made Aware"

The primary objective for this book is to raise awareness of the latest advances in developmental science and their implications for the varied practices and policies (ie, medical, educational, social, and economic) that touch young children, their families, and their communities. Specifically, we hope to raise awareness about

- **Epigenetics, developmental neuroscience, and intervention science.** Advances in these developmental sciences are forcing us to reconsider the early life origins of adult-manifest disease, and they are challenging us to do a better job of getting genomes, brains, and relationships right the first time, instead of constantly trying to repair, remediate, or fix seemingly intractable problems later.

- **The inadequacy of most models of disease and wellness.** Most models do not consider the dimension of time. Future models must incorporate the latest knowledge regarding the ongoing but cumulative dance between nurture and nature that governs genomic function, influences the wiring of the brain, and drives behavior not only in childhood but across the life span.

- **The advantages of the ecobiodevelopmental (EBD) model.** These are outlined in Chapter 5, but perhaps the most important advantage is that the EBD model replaces mind-body dualism with environmentally induced changes at the molecular, cellular, and behavioral levels. These changes are cumulative, are driving development over time and across the life span, and are later deemed as adaptive or maladaptive depending on the context.

- **The dangers of unmet deficiency needs (ie, physiology, safety, connection, and esteem).** These are all basic biological needs because, when they are unmet, they have the potential to induce the toxic stress responses that are known to alter genomic function and brain development. Unmet deficiency needs simply make it harder for children (and the adults who care for them) to self-actualize and to fulfill their potential.

- **The importance of relational health** and the capacity of safe, stable, and nurturing relationships to buffer early childhood adversity and toxic stress. Safe, stable, and nurturing relationships release the brake that toxic stress places on healthy, adaptive development, and they complement educational efforts to step on the gas by building new skills.

- **The many implications of the EBD model** for how we, as parents and caregivers, raise our children and how we, as pediatricians, neighbors, and policy makers, support other parents and caregivers as they nurture their children. As outlined in Part 2, a public health approach is needed to build relational health, eliminate barriers to relational health, and repair relational health once it has been strained. In addition to this vertical integration (ie, primary prevention, secondary interventions, and tertiary treatments), the public health approach needs to be integrated horizontally, breaking down silos between medicine, mental health, education, social services, and justice systems.

We believe that an understanding of this developmental biology and its implications for health, education, and social services is requisite knowledge for all professionals who aspire to make future generations better off than the previous ones. At the very least, we hope these important concepts will become standard fare for all medical students and pediatric trainees.

Our Dreams: "Every Child Must Be Made to Care"

We believe that the concepts presented in this book are potentially transformational, but translating these biologically grounded concepts into a better reality will require a political movement that transcends party lines and replaces narrow ideologies with a broader vision of how childhood adversity and relational health affect the well-being, educational success, and economic productivity of generations to come. At the moment, the political will to reframe health, education, social service, and economic policies based on science[4] and what we know about human skill formation is sorely lacking. Nevertheless, we dream of a "care-full" future, where

- **Our common biology transcends divisive politics.** Realizing that the threat of toxic stress is not bound by zip code, race, or wealth, politicians and policy makers of all persuasions embrace the important buffering capacity of relational health. Pending legislation and public policies are, therefore, viewed through the lens of relational health: Will these laws and policies promote safe, stable, and nurturing relationships, or will they make safe, stable, and nurturing relationships harder to achieve and sustain?
- **Developmental science informs efforts to close the disparities** in medical, educational, and economic outcomes that erode our collective identity and overall connectedness. All too often, discussions about disparities degenerate into debates about personal accountability versus equal opportunity. Developmental science reframes disparities as established threats to our collective relational health, but these threats are firmly grounded in our shared biology and distinctive ecologies. Developmental science offers the opportunity to narrow these widening disparities by promoting safe, stable, and nurturing relationships and supporting the early childhood ecologies that optimize human skill formation.
- **Safe, stable, and nurturing relationships are modeled, taught, practiced, and reinforced** through formalized social and emotional learning standards.[5-7] The social and emotional skills needed to form and sustain

safe, stable, and nurturing relationships are learned and absolutely necessary for wellness, educational success, and economic productivity. Formalized social and emotional learning standards are not about character formation or attempts to secularize morality; they are about helping children develop the foundational skills needed to be healthy and successful in the 21st century.[8]

- **Unmet deficiency needs are recognized as biological threats to relational health,** so the medical, educational, and social service sectors work collaboratively to ensure that all children (and their caregivers) have the opportunity to fulfill their potential and become the best possible versions of themselves.

- **Relational health is celebrated.** Efforts like Making Caring Common,[9] Start With Hello,[10] and No One Eats Alone[11] would no longer be necessary because efforts that reach out to the alienated and marginalized through random acts of kindness receive more media attention than divisiveness, escalating conflicts, and random acts of violence.

Pediatricians Must Lead the Way...

We believe in the transformational potential of the EBD model, and we firmly believe that pediatricians must take the lead in this work. But we must engage all our medical and nonmedical colleagues if tangible change and sustainable progress are to be achieved. Transitioning from a sick-care system to one that focuses on well care will require an almost monumental paradigm shift toward thinking developmentally and thinking ecologically, as well as dramatic changes in health care education and delivery.[12] Health care leaders need to understand that many of the chronic, noncommunicable diseases of adulthood are often manifestations of childhood adversity (adult-*manifest* diseases), and the allocation of resources must change if we intend to get at the root causes of many of our most intractable problems.

...But Everyone Has a Contribution to Make

Similar to the way that a toxic stress response might appear initially to be adaptive but prove to be harmful over time, disparities, inequities, marginalization, racism, and nationalism might empower the insecure with a sense of superiority and provide the fearful with an illusion of security. But we dream of a day when students of human development recognize all these divisions as intergenerational threats to relational health and our collective well-being. We dream of the day when a comprehensive, integrated public health approach is implemented, not only to address early childhood adversity and toxic stress but to proactively build, eliminate barriers to, and repair relational health. We believe such an approach has the best chance to translate what is known about human development into healthy children, nurturing families, and communities that care. Promoting lifelong health begins by nurturing wellness in childhood.

References

1. Fraser I, Grossman L, Kohan, A. Peace on Earth/Little Drummer Boy. Elstree Studios. London, United Kingdom: RCA Records; 1977

2. Winchell W. Walter Winchell in New York. *Naugatuck Daily News.* April 6, 1949. https://www.newspapers.com/newspage/33703223. Accessed March 1, 2018

3. Herring L. *Writing Begins with the Breath: Embodying Your Authentic Voice.* Boston, MA: Shambhala Publications Inc; 2007

4. Levitan D. *Not a Scientist: How Politicians Mistake, Misrepresent, and Utterly Mangle Science.* New York, NY: W.W. Norton & Company; 2017

5. Durlak JA, Weissberg RP, Dymnicki AB, Taylor RD, Schellinger KB. The impact of enhancing students' social and emotional learning: a meta-analysis of school-based universal interventions. *Child Dev.* 2011;82(1):405–432

6. Payton J, Weissberg RP, Durlak JA, et al. *The Positive Impact of Social and Emotional Learning for Kindergarten to Eighth-Grade Students: Findings From Three Scientific Reviews.* https://www.casel.org/wp-content/uploads/2016/06/the-positive-impact-of-social-and-emotional-learning-for-kindergarten-to-eighth-grade-students-executive-summary.pdf. Published December 2008. Accessed March 1, 2018

7. Collaborative for Academic, Social, and Emotional Learning (CASEL). What is SEL? http://www.casel.org/what-is-sel. Accessed March 1, 2018

8. Jana LA. *The Toddler Brain: Nurture the Skills Today that Will Shape Your Child's Tomorrow; the Surprising Science Behind Your Child's Development from Birth to Age 5.* Boston, MA: Da Capo Press; 2017

9. Harvard Graduate School of Education Making Caring Common Project. https://mcc.gse.harvard.edu. Accessed March 1, 2018

10. Sandy Hook Promise. Start with hello: promoting social inclusion and community connectedness. https://d3n8a8pro7vhmx.cloudfront.net/promise/pages/96/attachments/original/1442958562/Start_With_Hello.pdf?1442958562. Accessed March 1, 2018

11. Beyond Differences. Welcome to National No One Eats Alone Day! http://www.nooneeatsalone.org/welcome. Accessed March 1, 2018

12. Garner AS. Thinking developmentally: the next evolution in models of health. *J Dev Behav Pediatr.* 2016;37(7):579–584

Glossary of Terms, Concepts, and Abbreviations

AAP: Acronym for the American Academy of Pediatrics, a national organization of primary care pediatricians, pediatric medical subspecialists, and pediatric surgical specialists founded in 1930 and dedicated to the optimal physical, mental, and social health and well-being of infants, children, adolescents, and young adults.

ABC: Acronym for Attachment and Biobehavioral Catch-up, an evidence-based program of interventions designed by Mary Dozier, PhD, and colleagues to assist foster parents in nurturing children who have experienced disruptions in care and who exhibit disorganized attachments.

ACEs: Acronym for adverse childhood experiences. In the original ACE Study by Drs Vincent Felitti and Robert Anda, 10 categories of adversity were examined: emotional, physical, and sexual abuse; 5 measures of household dysfunction, including mother treated violently (intimate partner violence), household substance abuse, household mental illness, parental separation or divorce, and incarcerated household member; and emotional and physical neglect. Other investigators have applied the term ACEs to additional adversities known to affect child health, like poverty, neighborhood violence, and exposure to racism.

ACE score: The sum of the 10 different categories of ACEs experienced prior to the 18th birthday. To determine an individual's ACE score, see https://acestoohigh.com/got-your-ace-score. *See also* ACEs.

Adrenal cortex: The outer layer of the adrenal gland that sits above each kidney and responds to corticotropin with the release of cortisol. *See also* Corticotropin; Cortisol.

Adrenal medulla: The inner core of the adrenal gland that sits above each kidney and responds to activation of the sympathetic nervous system with the release of epinephrine and norepinephrine. *See also* Epinephrine; Norepinephrine.

Affiliative experiences: Events that promote early relational health; they are positive, affirming, and inclusive. Examples include interactions with engaged, attentive caregivers; access to health care professionals; quality early education services; and even ample opportunities to play with peers.

Allostasis: The body's active attempts to return to baseline (or equilibrium) after it has been disturbed. *See also* Behavioral allostasis.

Amygdala: An evolutionarily old brain structure that plays a major role in emotion processing and responses. It is the primary *on* switch for the body's stress response system. Generally speaking, it is larger and more powerful after sustained adversities, like growing up in an orphanage or being raised with a mother who experiences depression.

Apoptosis: Also known as *programmed cell death;* occurs in many of the neurons generated in utero, thereby eliminating any excess neurons.

Attachment: Bond that develops between young children and their adult caregivers. Depending on type of experiences that young children have with their primary caregivers, children might develop a secure, anxious-ambivalent, anxious-avoidant, or disorganized attachment. Safe, stable, and nurturing relationships promote secure attachments.

Axon: Part of a neuron that transmits electrical and chemical information to other cells, often over long distances. Myelinated axons transmit electrical signals faster than non-myelinated axons. Axons end in synapses with other cells.

Barker hypothesis: The proposal by British epidemiologist David J. P. Barker that intrauterine growth retardation, low birth weight, and preterm birth are causally related to the development of hypertension, coronary artery disease, and non–insulin-dependent diabetes mellitus in adulthood. When Barker proposed this hypothesis in 1990, he was largely ridiculed because there were no known biological mechanisms to explain how early experiences could become biologically embedded and affect health outcomes decades later. Today, we understand that epigenetic mechanisms are at play.

Behavioral allostasis: Behavioral attempts to return to baseline after the body has been disturbed. In the context of adversity, behavioral allostasis is manifest in the adoption of behaviors (eg, the Big 5) that transiently turn off the body's stress response. *See also* Allostasis; Big 5.

Big 5: 1) Overeating (a proxy for obesity), 2) promiscuity, and the use of 3) tobacco, 4) alcohol, and 5) illicit drugs. These are examples of behavioral allostasis in that they transiently turn off the body's stress response. But they are also maladaptive in the long run, as they are known risk factors for most of the adult-manifest, noncommunicable diseases associated with early childhood adversity.

Biomedical model: The physical, biological mechanisms of disease; excludes psychological, environmental, and social influences. It focuses on disorders of life and not disorders of living. It embraces reductionism and the idea that disease is frequently due to one physical etiology, like the mutation of a gene or an infection by a type of bacteria. It acknowledges mind-body dualism, which draws a distinction between the physical body (which is governed by biology) and the mind (which is governed by psychology, sociology, and free will). *See also* Biopsychosocial model; Ecobiodevelopmental (EBD) model.

Biopsychosocial model: The complex interactions between biological, psychological, and social factors that contribute to disease. It focuses on disorders and life and living and rejects mind-body dualism and the distinction between the body and the mind (because the mind arises from the functioning of the brain). *See also* Biomedical model; Ecobiodevelopmental (EBD) model.

Cellular plasticity: The brain's ability to form new synapses (synaptogenesis) in response to previous experiences. It is the equivalent of going from one person shouting to a stadium shouting. But most of the brain's cellular plasticity is waning by the time children reach kindergarten. *See also* Plasticity; Synaptic plasticity; Synaptogenesis.

Child-parent psychotherapy (CPP): An evidence-based, psychoanalytic approach advanced by Alicia Lieberman, PhD, and others to treating dysfunctional parent-child relationships based on the theory that the parent has unresolved conflicts with previous relationships.

Circle of security: A parent education and psychotherapy intervention that promotes developmentally appropriate interactions between the parent and child to promote a more organized and secure attachment.

Communities That Care (CTC): An evidence-based approach that uses social development theory to address a wide array of adolescent problem behaviors, including substance abuse, violence, truancy, and teen pregnancy. An integral element of this approach is clear, consistent messaging about social norms and expectations.

Corticotropin: Hormone released by the pituitary in response to corticotropin-releasing hormone (CRH) that stimulates the adrenal cortex to release cortisol. Also referred to as adrenocorticotropic hormone (ACTH). *See also* Corticotropin-releasing hormone; Cortisol.

Corticotropin-releasing hormone: Produced in the hypothalamus and triggers cells in the anterior pituitary to secrete corticotropin. *See also* Corticotropin.

Cortisol: A glucocorticoid steroid hormone produced in the adrenal cortex in response to corticotropin. *See also* Corticotropin.

Deficiency needs: According to Abraham Maslow, PhD, sources of motivation. When unmet, deficiency needs, like physiologic needs (eg, food, water, sleep) and the need to feel safe, connected, and competent, inhibit the innate growth needs, like the drive to self-actualize or to transcend one's experience (see Box 6-1). *See also* Growth needs; Meta-motivation; Motivation; Self-actualize.

Dendrites: Parts of neurons that are covered in synapses and receive information from other cells. The larger the dendritic arbor, the more synapses and the more information that neuron receives and processes. *See also* Neurons; Synapse.

Developmental origins of health and disease: Interdisciplinary field of study that examines the fetal and developmental underpinnings of disease and health. Although originally focused on nutritional concerns, the field has grown to include all aspects of early human development in relation to chronic diseases later in life.

DNA: Chemical that encodes genetic information within the sequence of its base pairs. Chromosomes are made of DNA and proteins, like histones, that organize the DNA and determine which parts of the DNA are transcribed into RNA. *See also* RNA.

DNA methylation: An epigenetic mechanism that adds a methyl ($-CH_3$) group directly to the DNA and generally turns the expression of that gene off.

Dyadic dance: Serve and return interactions between young children and their adult caregivers.

Ecobiodevelopmental (EBD) model: Builds on the biomedical and biopsychosocial models by adding the dimension of time. The EBD model argues that the environment becomes biologically embedded and the ongoing but cumulative dance between the environment (nurture) and the genome (nature) drives development not only in childhood but across the life span. It rejects mind-body dualism, arguing that experience-induced alterations at the molecular, cellular, and behavioral levels will prove to be adaptive or maladaptive over time depending on the context. *See also* Biomedical model; Biopsychosocial model.

Epigenetics: Study of functionally relevant (and potentially heritable) chemical modifications to DNA and associated genomic proteins that do not involve a change in the DNA nucleotide sequence.

Epigenome: Entirety of the chemical modifications of the genome and associated genomic proteins that alter gene expression without changing the nucleotide sequence. *See also* Genome.

Epinephrine: Also known as adrenalin; a hormone secreted by the adrenal medulla in response to activation of the sympathetic nervous system. *See also* Adrenal medulla.

Family-centered pediatric medical home (FCPMH): The American Academy of Pediatrics defines the *medical home* as a model of delivering primary care that is accessible, continuous, comprehensive, family centered, coordinated, compassionate, and culturally effective. It does not refer to a specific building but to the integrated services provided by a team of professionals and led by a pediatrician.

Genome: Complete DNA sequences, supporting proteins, and associated chemicals comprising the entirety of the hereditary information.

Genotype: Genetic constitution of an organism or cell; also refers to the specific set of alleles inherited at a locus (see Figure 3-1). *See also* Phenotype.

Glucocorticoid receptor: Also known as *NR3C1* (nuclear receptor subfamily 3, group C, member 1); the receptor for cortisol and other glucocorticoids. Glucocorticoid receptors in the hypothalamus and pituitary play an important role in the negative feedback loop that downregulates the generation of more cortisol. *See also* Cortisol; Glucocorticoids.

Glucocorticoids: A class of steroid hormones. Cortisol is a glucocorticoid, as are several medicines like prednisone and methylprednisolone. *See also* Cortisol.

Gray matter: The largely non-myelinated areas of the brain. Because axons are wrapped in myelin and myelin appears white on a cross section of the brain, areas of the brain that appear gray (and not white) consist primarily of cell bodies and dendrites. In general, the thicker the gray matter that covers the surface of the brain, the more cell bodies, dendrites, and synapses are present. Hence, the process of synaptic pruning results in a thinning of the gray matter. *See also* White matter.

Growth needs: According to Abraham Maslow, sources of meta-motivation, or the innate drive to self-actualize and to transcend one's experience, that are manifest once one's deficiency needs have been met (see Box 6-1). *See also* Deficiency needs; Meta-motivation; Motivation; Self-actualize.

Hippocampus: Structure in the brain that plays an important role in learning and memory, but it can be inhibited by stress and an activated amygdala. Conversely, the hippocampus and prefrontal cortex are potential *off* switches for the amygdala and the body's stress response system. *See also* Amygdala; Prefrontal cortex.

Histone acetylation: Epigenetic mechanism that places acetyl groups ($-CH_2-CH_3$) on histones, generally enhancing DNA accessibility and turning on the expression of genes.

Histones: Structural proteins associated with the DNA molecule.

Horizontal integration: Public health approach that cuts across traditional silos and includes not only health care but the educational, social service, and juvenile justice systems (see Figure 6-1). *See also* Vertical integration.

Hypothalamic-pituitary-adrenal (HPA) axis: Ability of the hypothalamus to trigger (via corticotropin-releasing hormone) the release of corticotropin from the pituitary. Corticotropin then acts on the adrenal cortex to release glucocorticoids like cortisol. *See also* Corticotropin; Corticotropin-releasing hormone; Cortisol; Hypothalamus.

Hypothalamus: Structure in the brain that functions as a link between the nervous and endocrine systems. It plays a major role in monitoring and regulating vital functions like body temperature, thirst, hunger, sleep, and attachment behaviors.

Imprinting: Process by which maternally and paternally derived chromosomes are uniquely chemically modified, leading to differential expression of a certain gene or genes on those chromosomes depending on their parental origin.

Life course science: Retrospective epidemiological research and prospective interventional studies that look for associations between childhood experiences and outcomes as an adolescent or adult.

Limbic system: Set of structures in the brain, including the amygdala, hypothalamus, and hippocampus, that play an important role in emotion processing and regulation. *See also* Amygdala; Hippocampus; Hypothalamus.

Meta-motivation: According to Abraham Maslow, the innate drive to self-actualize or to transcend one's experience that is manifest once one's deficiency needs have been met (see Box 6-1). *See also* Deficiency needs; Growth needs; Motivation; Self-actualize.

Mind-body dualism: The idea that the mind and body are distinct and separate entities.

Motivation: According to Abraham Maslow, the innate drive to meet one's deficiency needs (see Box 6-1). *See also* Deficiency needs; Growth needs; Meta-motivation; Self-actualize.

Motivational interviewing: Counseling method that engages the patient in a trusting and respectful working relationship, focuses the relationship on making progress toward shared goals or objectives, evokes the client's own motivations and strategies for change while remaining hopeful and confident, and plans, in conjunction with the client, specific actions that the patient has committed to taking. In motivational interviewing, the counselor does a lot of reflective listening to highlight the patient's internal goals, motivations, and plans for change and to assist the patient in resolving his or her ambivalence to change.

Myelination: Wrapping of axons by oligodendrocytes, thereby increasing the speed of axonal transmission. In general, myelination is a measure of structural maturity, so the more myelinated an area is, the more mature it is. In some areas of the brain, like the prefrontal cortex, myelination is not complete until 24 years of age.

Neurogenesis: Generation or birth of new neurons. With a few notable exceptions, neurogenesis occurs primarily in utero.

Neurons: Electrically active cells in the brain that rapidly process information. Neurons receive chemical and electrical information along their dendrites, and they transmit electrical and chemical information along their axons, which terminate in synapses with other cells. *See also* Axon; Dendrites; Synapse.

Noncoding RNA (ncRNA): Messenger RNA that is not translated into protein; generally comes in long or short (microRNA) forms. Because ncRNAs affect genetic expression, they are an additional epigenetic mechanism.

Norepinephrine: Also known as noradrenalin; a hormone secreted by the adrenal medulla in response to activation of the sympathetic nervous system.

Parent-child interaction therapy (PCIT): Evidence-based intervention by Sheila Eyberg, PhD, and colleagues to change the patterns of parent-child interactions to improve the parent-child relationship.

Pediatric way: Traditional role that pediatricians have played in translating the latest advances in science into not only clinical practice but the public policies that improve the health and well-being of children, their families, and their communities.

Phenotype: Observable physical and biochemical characteristics of the expression of a gene; the clinical presentation of an individual with a particular genotype (see Figure 3-1). *See also* Genotype.

Plasticity: Ability of the brain and genome to alter their function in response to previous experiences. *See also* Cellular plasticity; Synaptic plasticity.

Positive stress response: Activation of the body's stress response system that is brief, infrequent, and mild in intensity. Examples include the typical changes that are faced and overcome by children every day (eg, expressing one's needs verbally, separation anxiety, minor/incidental traumas). Positive stress responses are more likely if an adversity is buffered by the presence of safe, stable, and nurturing relationships. A positive stress response is not the absence of adversity, but it reflects an ability to cope with adversity in a healthy, adaptive manner, thereby building confidence and competence in the face of future adversity. *See also* Tolerable stress response; Toxic stress response.

Prefrontal cortex: Evolutionarily newer brain structure that has been called the "seat of humanity" because it allows for the abstract thought, planning, emotion regulation, and control of attention necessary for humans to imagine, create, and collaborate. Along with the hippocampus, the prefrontal cortex is a potential *off* switch for the amygdala and the body's stress response system. Generally speaking, it is thinner and less powerful after sustained adversities, like growing up in an orphanage or in a family that is impoverished. *See also* Amygdala; Hippocampus.

Pruning: Elimination of excess synapses; strongly influenced by experiences and the neuronal activity generated by experiences (ie, "If you don't use it, you lose it").

Reach Out and Read: Nonprofit organization and early literacy program; developed by pediatricians Dr Barry Zuckerman and Dr Robert Needlman, and educators Jean Nigro, Kathleen MacLean, and Kathleen Fitzgerald-Rice at Boston City Hospital in 1989. Reach Out and Read provides age-appropriate books and encourages parents to regularly read to and interact with their children to support school readiness and healthy attachments.

Relational health: Ability to form and maintain safe, stable, and nurturing relationships; an important predictor of lifelong health.

Relational mode: Ability of safe, stable, and nurturing relationships to inhibit the amygdala and promote the prefrontal cortex and hippocampus. Relational mode does not refer to a static state but to one pole of an ongoing, dynamic flux with survival mode, based on current context and previous experiences (see Figure 4-3). *See also* Survival mode.

Resilience: Ability to respond to adversity in a healthy, adaptive manner; reflects a set of skills that can be modeled, nurtured, taught, and practiced, often in the context of safe, stable, and nurturing relationships.

Restorative justice: Efforts that repair the harm that occurs with unjust behaviors, as opposed to efforts that simply punish those who have acted unjustly (retributive justice). Typically, restorative justice allows victims and offenders to mediate a restitution agreement that is satisfactory to both parties. In this way, the victims play an active role in communicating with and understanding the offenders, and the offenders have the chance to take responsibility for their actions, identify steps that might prevent offending behaviors in the future, and redeem themselves in the eyes of the victims and the community. *See also* Retributive justice.

Retributive justice: Efforts that simply punish those who have acted unjustly, as opposed to efforts that focus on repairing the harm that occurs with unjust behaviors (restorative justice). With retributive justice, the state holds offenders accountable for their actions by imposing punishments that are deemed to be in proportion to the offense. In this way, the victims play a limited, if any, role in communicating with or understanding the offenders, and the offenders have limited, if any, opportunities for rehabilitation or to identify steps that might prevent offending behaviors in the future. *See also* Restorative justice.

RNA: Synthesized from the DNA template (see Figure 3-1); contains the sugar ribose instead of deoxyribose, which is present in DNA. Four forms exist: messenger (mRNA), transfer (tRNA), ribosomal (rRNA), and noncoding (ncRNA). *See also* DNA; Noncoding RNA (ncRNA).

Self-actualize: According to Abraham Maslow, there is an innate drive or meta-motivation to self-actualize—to use one's capabilities and fulfill one's potential—but it is only manifest once one's deficiency needs have been met (see Box 6-1). *See also* Deficiency needs; Growth needs; Meta-motivation; Motivation.

Survival mode: Ability of significant childhood adversity to promote the amygdala and inhibit the prefrontal cortex and hippocampus. Survival mode does not refer to a static state but to one pole of an ongoing, dynamic flux with relational mode, based on current context and previous experiences (see Figure 4-3). *See also* Relational mode.

Sympatho-adrenomedullary (SAM) pathway: Neurons of the hypothalamospinal tract that activate the sympathetic nervous system, which, in turn, stimulates the adrenal medulla to release epinephrine and norepinephrine. *See also* Adrenal medulla.

Synapse: Terminal end of a neuron's axon where chemical information is rapidly shared with another cell, typically the dendrite of another neuron. *See also* Axon; Dendrites; Neurons.

Synaptic plasticity: Changes in the strength of the connection between 2 neurons. It is the equivalent of turning up the volume in a speaker and is thought to be a lifelong form of learning. *See also* Cellular plasticity; Plasticity.

Synaptogenesis: Generation of new synapses between neurons in the brain. In early childhood, there are more than 1 million new synapses forming per second. Synaptogenesis is strongly influenced by experiences and the neuronal activity generated by experiences (ie, "neurons that fire together, wire together"). *See also* Synapse.

Transcription: Process of synthesizing messenger RNA from DNA (see Figure 3-1). *See also* Translation.

Translation: Process of synthesizing an amino acid sequence (protein product) from RNA (see Figure 3-1). *See also* Transcription.

Tolerable stress response: Activation of the body's stress response system that is longer lasting, more frequent, and moderate to severe in intensity (eg, death of a parent, moving away from trusted social supports). Unlike positive stress responses, tolerable stress responses are less likely to build confidence or competence, but they are also less likely to trigger the potentially permanent changes induced by toxic stress responses. Tolerable stress responses are more likely if an adversity is buffered by the presence of safe, stable, and nurturing relationships. *See also* Positive stress response; Toxic stress response.

Toxic stress response: Activation of the body's stress response system that is sustained, frequent, and severe in intensity (eg, adverse childhood experiences). Toxic stress responses are more likely if an adversity is *not* buffered by the presence of safe, stable, and nurturing relationships. Toxic stress responses trigger changes at the molecular, cellular, and behavioral levels that might be initially adaptive (eg, behavioral allostasis) but prove to be maladaptive in the long term (eg, Big 5). *See also* ACEs; Behavioral allostasis; Big 5; Positive stress response; Tolerable stress response.

Vagal nerve: Tenth cranial nerve. As part of the parasympathetic nervous system, it helps to control bodily functions like heart rate, blood pressure, and respiration by countering the effects of the sympatho-adrenomedullary pathway and the sympathetic nervous system. *See also* Sympatho-adrenomedullary (SAM) pathway.

Vertical integration: Public health approach that includes primary, universal preventions to promote wellness; secondary, targeted interventions for those deemed to be at risk for poor outcomes; and tertiary, evidence-based treatments for the symptomatic (see Figure 6-1). *See also* Horizontal integration.

White matter: Heavily myelinated regions seen in cross sections of the brain. Myelin is a fatty substance within the oligodendrocytes that wrap around axons and speed up the rate of axonal transmission. Because myelin appears white, the central regions of the brain that appear white contain large numbers of myelinated axons. *See also* Gray matter.

Appendix B

Abridged, Amended Version of the AAP *Blueprint for Children*

Prior to the 2016 US presidential election, the American Academy of Pediatrics (AAP) published *Blueprint for Children: How the Next President Can Build a Foundation for a Healthy Future.* In this document, the AAP outlined general goals and specific policy recommendations for healthy children, secure families, and strong communities. The AAP argued that these goals and recommendations are necessary for the United States to remain a leading nation. Many of these goals and recommendations are included, often word for word, in the following abridged and amended version. But here, the focus is on building *healthy, resilient children* through *strong families* and *communities that care,* and so we have expanded on some of the recommendations in the *Blueprint for Children.* These policy recommendations are grounded in the developmental science discussed throughout this book. By thinking developmentally, applying a public health approach, and nurturing wellness in childhood, we are promoting lifelong health.

Building Healthy, Resilient Children

Goals

1. All children have their essential needs (ie, physiologic, safety, connection, and self-esteem) met.
2. All children, regardless of their immigration status, are covered by affordable health care coverage that is comprehensive and includes pediatric-specific and 2-generational benefits.
3. All children receive primary care in a medical home that is family centered.
4. All children have access to needed subspecialty pediatric care and mental health services.

Potential Policy Objectives

1. Ensure that all public and private health plans for children offer a comprehensive, well-defined, and pediatric-specific essential health benefits package that includes a broad range of services, including evidence-based programs that promote relational health (eg, Reach Out and Read, home visiting programs), eliminate barriers to relational health (eg, screening for and addressing child and/or parental mental health problems; Health Leads; Well-child Care Visit, Evaluation, Community Resources, Advocacy, Referral, Education [WE CARE]; iScreen; medicolegal partnerships), and repair relational health (eg, Attachment and Biobehavioral Catch-up; child-parent psychotherapy; parent-child interactive therapy).

2. Improve financing for high-quality, team-based medical and mental health care delivered in a family-centered medical home that incorporates Bright Futures guidelines and Early and Periodic Screening, Diagnosis, and Treatment services.

3. Continue to support the Children's Health Insurance Program.

4. Improve access to Medicaid services by simplifying eligibility processes, reducing bureaucratic barriers to care, and streamlining enrollment, including linkages to other programs like nutrition assistance.

5. Ensure that Medicaid and other key entitlement programs for children are not subject to payment caps, block grants, or other structural harms.

6. Address inequities between Medicaid and Medicare payment so children have better access to health care professionals and services.

7. Safeguard the access of military families to appropriate supports by strengthening services provided through TRICARE.

8. Promote maternal and reproductive health care services.

9. Offer loan repayment programs to pediatricians and subspecialists who work in underserved areas or care for a significant share of low-income patients.

10. Revise confidentiality rules to promote collaboration among the medical home, the educational community, and social services and help ensure that children's essential needs are met.

Building Strong Families

As pediatric clinicians, we can and must do more to support families as they nurture within their children the behaviors and skills necessary for healthy and productive life course trajectories.

Goals

1. All the goals outlined previously for building healthy, resilient children, because today's children will parent the next generation of families.
2. All families have access to resources that support relational health and the adoption of positive parenting practices.
3. All families have opportunities for work that provide a stable and adequate income and family-friendly benefits, and those opportunities are not tied to their eligibility for programs like Medicaid.
4. All families have safe and secure housing.
5. All families have affordable and safe child care.
6. All families have access to adequate, healthy, and nutritious food throughout the year.

Potential Policy Objectives

1. Increase opportunities to lift families out of poverty, including raising the minimum wage, offering job training, strengthening the earned income tax credit and child tax credit, expanding the Temporary Assistance for Needy Families program, strengthening the Supplemental Nutrition Assistance Program, and expanding family and medical leave.
2. Make significant investments to ensure access to affordable and high-quality child care for all families, including support for the Office of Child Care in the Administration for Children and Families and the Child Care and Development Block Grant Act.
3. Improve public support for affordable and safe housing, including expansion of federal rental assistance, to end family homelessness, reduce housing instability, and help struggling families to afford their rent.
4. Expand and continue programs for at-risk parents, such as the Maternal, Infant, and Early Childhood Home Visiting Program, to identify and connect parents with community services that treat parental depression or substance abuse, mitigate other precipitants of toxic stress, and promote child well-being.
5. Improve the child welfare system to prevent child abuse and neglect, better serve vulnerable children and their families, and ensure that children and caregivers have access to coordinated, high-quality, trauma-informed health and social services.
6. Protect and strengthen federal nutrition programs for children and families—especially pregnant mothers—including breastfeeding promotion; Supplemental Nutritional Assistance Program; the Special Supplemental Nutrition Program for Women, Infants, and Children;

the Child and Adult Care Food Program; the National School Lunch Program and School Breakfast Program; and the Summer Food Service Program.

7. Increase peer and community social supports for young families through programs like Centering Pregnancy, Centering Parenting, and Legacy for Children.

Building Communities That Care

As pediatric clinicians, we recognize the positive effect that strong and secure families have on their children. But we also recognize that is it far easier to build strong and secure families when they live in communities that care.

Goals

1. All the goals outlined previously for building strong families, because families make communities. Much like individuals, it may be hard for families to think relationally when they are in survival mode. When families are safe and secure, they may be more likely to engage in how their community nurtures and cares for other families (eg, voting, advocating, simply setting the tone).
2. Communities are safe from violence and free of environmental hazards (eg, lead).
3. Communities provide high-quality early education programs.
4. Communities support public health systems that protect children from infectious diseases and support maternal and child health.
5. Communities respond effectively when disasters and public health emergencies occur.
6. Communities actively promote relational health by denouncing racism, hatred, and oppression and actively supporting the disadvantaged within their midst.

Potential Policy Objectives

1. Conduct federally funded research to build the evidence base for a public health response to violence, including research on gun violence coordinated by the Centers for Disease Control and Prevention (CDC).
2. Expand efforts to ensure that firearms do not get into the wrong hands by passing comprehensive, commonsense gun violence prevention measures, such as banning assault weapons and improving background checks.

3. Increase the number of children in prekindergarten education and improve access to proven, high-quality early learning programs, such as Head Start and Early Head Start.

4. Strengthen laws and programs to ensure that children live in clean environments, including clean air and water and safe housing, through US Environmental Protection Agency air and water quality standards and US Department of Housing and Urban Development public housing standards; the recent banning of smoking is a good example.

5. Address aging and outdated infrastructure and its effects on lead in the water.

6. Strengthen programs to provide low-income neighborhoods with resources to ensure that all children and adolescents have access to safe and desirable opportunities for play and active lifestyles.

7. Bolster efforts to reduce the burden of preventable infectious disease by supporting vaccination efforts at the CDC and the Health Resources and Services Administration.

8. Ensure that biodefense and public health programs at the CDC, US Department of Health and Human Services Assistant Secretary for Preparedness and Response, and Maternal and Child Health Bureau are fully funded and that they prioritize the needs of children before, during, and after natural and human-made disasters.

9. Increase support for formalized social and emotional learning in schools.

10. Expand evidence-based programs that promote restorative justice.

Index

Page numbers followed by an *f,* a *t,* or a *b* denote a figure, a table, or a box, respectively.

A

R

Raising Human Beings, 96
Reach Out and Read program, 88, 121,
    136
Reagan, Ronald, 140
Relational health
    active promotion of, 119–121
    barriers to, 113–119, 134
    benefits of, 140
    case studies of, 119–120
    celebrating of, 146
    clinical vignettes on, 110–111,
        113–115
    community support for, 94–98, 138
    corporal punishment, effects of, 112
    definition of, 47
    importance of, 144
    parental barriers to, 83, 87
    poverty, effects of, 118
    repairing of, 110–113
    two-generational approaches to,
        87–88
    universal interventions for promotion
        of, 120–121
    unmet deficiency needs, effect of, 146
Relationships
    safe, stable, and nurturing. *See* Safe,
        stable, and nurturing relationships
        (SSNRs)
    therapeutic, 109
Research, 122–123
Resilience, 79, 136
Respect, 112
Richmond, Julius, 54*f,* 139–140
Roosevelt, Theodore, 105, 109

S

Safe, stable, and nurturing relationships
        (SSNRs)
    barriers to creation of, 83
    biological needs met through, 76, 83
    childhood adversity buffered by, 16
    deficiency needs met through, 134

ecobiodevelopmental model
    promotion of, 109
good-enough parenting based on, 77, 83
parental adverse childhood
    experiences, effect of, 84
parental provision of, 83, 86, 91
poverty, effects of, 87
self-actualization through, 76
social determinants of health, effect
    of, 117
teaching of, 145–146
toxic stress affected by, 46–47, 47*f,* 56,
    109, 144
Safety needs
    description of, 72*b,* 72–73, 73–74*t*
    of parents, 84
    unmet, community resources for, 92
SAM pathway. *See*
        Sympatho-adrenomedullary
        (SAM) pathway
Self-actualization
    deficiency needs as barrier to, 73*t,* 75,
        78, 82
    description of, 71
    good-enough parenting, effects on, 82
    in Maslow's hierarchy of needs, 71–72,
        74*t*
    of parents, 84
Self-esteem
    description of, 72*b,* 73–74*t*
    unmet needs for, 93
Sexual abuse, 4, 6
Shonkoff, Jack, 19
Sick-care system, 58
Smith, Walter Wellesley "Red," 143
Smoking, 7–8
Social determinants of health, 68, 71, 87,
    117–118, 134
Social development theory, 96
Social isolation, 86
Social referencing, 120–121
Social strategy, for advocacy, 139–140
Spanking, 112